CW00509259

Children without Language

Children without Language
From Dysphasia to Autism

Laurent Danon-Boileau

Translated from the French by
James Grieve

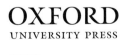
UNIVERSITY PRESS

2006

OXFORD
UNIVERSITY PRESS

Oxford University Press, Inc., publishes works that further
Oxford University's objective of excellence
in research, scholarship, and education.

Oxford   New York
Auckland   Cape Town   Dar es Salaam   Hong Kong   Karachi
Kuala Lumpur   Madrid   Melbourne   Mexico City   Nairobi
New Delhi   Shanghai   Taipei   Toronto

With offices in
Argentina   Austria   Brazil   Chile   Czech Republic   France   Greece
Guatemala   Hungary   Italy   Japan   Poland   Portugal   Singapore
South Korea   Switzerland   Thailand   Turkey   Ukraine   Vietnam

English translation © 2006 by Oxford University Press, Inc.

Ouvrage publié avec le concours du Ministère français chargé de la culture-Centre national
du livre. This translation is published with the support of the French Ministry of Culture-Centre
national du livre. Additional support provided by the Laboratory for the Study of the Acquisition
and Pathology of Language in Children, (LEAPLE, UMR 8606) Paris, France

Originally published in French as *Des enfants sans langage : De la dysphasie à l'autisme*
© Odile Jacob, January 2002

Published by Oxford University Press, Inc.
198 Madison Avenue, New York, New York 10016

www.oup.com

Oxford is a registered trademark of Oxford University Press

All rights reserved. No part of this publication may be reproduced,
stored in a retrieval system, or transmitted, in any form or by any means,
electronic, mechanical, photocopying, recording, or otherwise,
without the prior permission of Oxford University Press.

Library of Congress Cataloging-in-Publication Data
Danon-Boileau, Laurent, 1946–
[Enfants sans langage. English]
Children without language : from dysphasia to autism / by Laurent Danon-Boileau;
translated from the French by James Grieve.
p.   cm.
"Originally published in French as Des enfants sans langage."
Includes bibliographical references.
ISBN-13 978-0-19-517502-8
ISBN 0-19-517502-6
1. Language disorders in children.   2. Communicative disorders in children.   I. Title.
RF496.L35D3613   2005
618.92'855—dc22   2004029456

9 8 7 6 5 4 3 2 1

Printed in the United States of America
on acid-free paper

Contents

Part III Some Cases

Part IV Theoretical Foundations

Acknowledgments

First and foremost, I wish to thank my publisher, Odile Jacob, for her support. I must also express gratitude to the following colleagues, each of them a friend or a relative, for the many different ways in which they helped me either in working with the children or in the thinking that led to this book: Dr. J. Angelergues, M.-F. Bresson, M. Brigaudiot, C. Cahen-Salvador, C. Danon-Boileau, Dr. H. Danon-Boileau, M. Desgens, Professor R. Diatkine, J.-L. Fidel, Professor F. François, M. Garboua, Dr. G. Lucas, Dr. M. Ody, Dr. D. Morel, Professor M.-A. Morel, A. Maupas, A. Morgenstern, N. Parent, Dr. A. Philippe, V. Picchi, S. Robel, and M. Vassal.

I offer special thanks to my translator, James Grieve, and to my editor at Oxford University Press, Jennifer Rappaport. Their care and competence, their interest in the book, and the friendly relations that have developed between us through working together on this English version of my text make it much more than just a translation of the French edition. I am glad to express my gratitude and my profound indebtedness to both of them. The process of textual transformation for an English-speaking readership was also greatly helped by Virginia Picchi, to whom I am extremely grateful.

The author can be contacted at the following email address: danon@ext. jussieu.fr

Translator's Note

Where the French uses *il* (literally "he" or even "it"), as it often does, to refer to the antecedent *un enfant* ("a child," i.e., the masculine noun but of epicene reference), this translation will at times alternate between "he" and "she."

Children without Language

Introduction

Ways to Language

By the age of two or three, most children in the world have learned to talk. Not all of them, though: about 10 percent have what are called "communication and language problems." Fortunately, many such children will overcome these problems without great difficulty, though they may require the assistance of a speech therapist. There is, however, a minority—how many is difficult to estimate—who remain more profoundly affected. Some of them suffer from acute hearing disorders or even minor brain damage. The pathology in such cases is straightforward, if severe. But there are other children who, for reasons that may be a complete mystery, never speak at all. There may be whole range of different causes, such as language disorders or communication disorders, or both. The diagnosis may be imprecise, but the choice usually comes down to profound dysphasia (sometimes also called audimutism) or autism.

I am a professor of general linguistics and language pathology at the Sorbonne and a psychoanalyst, and these are the children I have been working with over the past fifteen years. The very first requirement of such work is to abide scrupulously by the old injunction *primum non nocere*: every therapist must endeavor not to harm the patient. In these cases, not harming entails being aware of the need to wait. There are times when the waiting can be protracted: some of these children can take three or four years before they start to speak. Regular monitoring of the progress made can be very instructive for the theorist. One learns how diverse reality can be, for even if two individuals are affected by the same disorder, the differences between them remain essential. Each case evolves in its own particular manner. When progress starts to happen, it can be this very particularity that helps one to understand the sequence of possible causes and the meaning of certain signs. It also brings out the factors that have enabled this or that child to accede to language. Not that more general considerations are ruled out, for different cases can have common features. The history of each case is like a metaphor or a myth for the birth of all language: it lets one see how all human beings must be able to invent their own idea of another person, the world, the use of signs, or their own thought processes, in order to be equipped to take part in the interplay of verbal communication. This gives food for thought in linguistics, psychoanalysis, and cognitive science, three points of view that will be seen to intertwine throughout my thinking on this subject.

As I write, I shall make clear the general principles that underlie my practice. However, I have neither the ability nor the desire to provide a cast-iron model of all developmental disorders in the fields of communication and language. I am a linguist and a psychoanalyst, with some knowledge of cognition and neuropsychology. It is certainly not my intention to bring about a synthesis of these fields. Instead of synthesizing, I am trying to look at the way each of these theoretical fields can help me understand the clinical facts I am confronted with. My intention is not to provide a definitive synthetic vision of language and communication disorders in children. This book is merely an attempt to build bridges between theories on the basis of clinical observations. What I really want is to show the possible links between positions held in totally discrete areas of knowledge, such as psychoanalysis and cognition, and to point out certain similarities to which proponents of these different theories seem to be blind. My main concern is to analyze and compare the various approaches and hypotheses on how communication is organized and how it breaks down.

My thinking is rooted in particular clinical events. In discussing each case, one of my aims will be to show how some fact observed during treatment contradicts the stereotype of the "notional toddler" we all have in our heads and why we must resist the notion that a child's progress in language is as straightforward and sequential as climbing a flight of stairs. Usually, it is more like the gradual taking shape of a picture on photosensitive paper, as the pigment begins to appear in the developing fluid tinged by the red glow of the darkroom. The shape forms and firms at different parts that are more exposed, without any of them being a necessary preliminary to the formation of any of the others. Attentiveness to each child's particularities makes one aware of the unpredictable diversity of the ways that lead to language. Unfortunately, it too often happens that our pre-conceived notion of progression by stages makes us think we know what a child in difficulty is capable of, on the basis of our assumptions about what the same child is incapable of. This can explain our propensity not to recognize the incongruous aptitudes of such children, despite the fact that clinical observation keeps bringing them to our attention.

In questioning the accepted model of the development of language and communication, I also hope to broach more general considerations, such as the effect of the power of language on an individual's way of being him- (or her-) self. In inspecting a particular disorder, I also investigate how much of it comes from a defect in the cerebral mechanism and how much from psychic origins, including the creative processes of thought and af-fect. In doing so, I am well aware of the danger of falling between three stools. However, to do the opposite is no less risky. Seeing things from a single point of view may well make them appear more coherent, but it also distorts them.

Obviously, when it is necessary to describe my ways as a therapist, I shall endeavor to be as precise and to the point as possible. As will be seen, I have no miracle method up my sleeve. What I do describe is more like a way of interacting and being interested, a way of relating, of being available, so as to keep a range of possible expectations open. It is impor-tant to do this without being too bothered or bored. It is a manner that is required of me in part by the needs of those I am dealing with, who hap-pen to be children who not only do not speak but who also have no facil-ity in communicating through facial expressions, gesture, or movement. But it also comes in part from who I am. The fact is that, as in all thera-peutic encounters but much more markedly in dealing with these par-ticular children, you have to make do with what you are and with what you feel. And the main thing one feels is uneasiness. There are times, for-tunately, when uneasiness turns to pleasure. Since I need a name for this therapeutic practice, I have come up with "psychoanalytic semiotherapy." I am, of course, convinced that, just as Monsieur Jourdain in Molière's *Le bourgeois gentilhomme* had been an unwitting speaker of prose for forty years, there was many a practitioner of semiotherapy before I came along.

In broad terms, this book represents a continuation of an earlier study of mine, published in 1995 with the title *L'Enfant qui ne disait rien* (trans-lated as *The Silent Child*, Oxford, 2001). The intervening years and fur-ther discussion have led me to more accurate definitions of some of the ideas presented in that book. I have given up some of my points of view, and I have worked out new ones. Most important, I have undertaken the salutary if painful exercise of setting limits to a therapeutic method. When *L'Enfant qui ne disait rien* appeared, most of the children who had been entrusted to me as patients up till then had progressed satisfactorily. They had language difficulties, and there were some with communication disorders, but once the link with others was established, it remained unbroken. They responded to their name and were quite willing to join me in pushing toy cars back and forth. At times their eye contact was evasive, but you could catch their eye, and they eventually smiled and pointed at objects that interested them. They could also tie their own shoelaces and hold a pencil. To most intents and purposes, they were kids much like other kids. Except, of course, that they said nothing. When the book came out, some parents whose children were still not speaking came to see me, among them some who reproached me roundly for my incompetence. Despite my best efforts, their children could hardly communicate, even by signs or movement. So gradually I found myself entertaining other aspects of child pathology. Autism and/or childhood psychosis seemed to be the sum total of possible diagnoses. These children were devoid of any desire to relate. They were unwilling to let anyone join in their activity and even more unwilling to join in anyone else's. They were either totally withdrawn or in a more worrying state of intense agitation. The slightest attempt at an approach to them, however unobtrusive, led only to a more marked distancing on their part. In addition, I became aware of something I had read about but that I had never really experienced for myself. I had always taken it for granted that the ability to speak went hand in hand with good nonverbal communication. This is simply not true: proficiency in language is no guarantee of effective communication. Though communication disorders are usually found in children devoid of language, they also occur in children who can speak. What these children say is a little off the point; their way of speaking is awkward, as though not belonging to them; and the words they use are like things thrown in to disrupt communication. Any exchange with them quickly turns to confusion. This is something I shall come back to as I describe the clinical sessions.

Generally speaking, when one considers communication disorders from a diagnostic perspective, things become quite complicated. For one thing, theoretical positions diverge from one another. More importantly, there is the fact that, when one is in the presence of a child, it is rather difficult to distinguish between symptoms that may well prove to be lasting and others that may wane. Very often, the available diagnostic categories resemble a net whose mesh is not fine enough to catch anything capable of giving a useful focus to therapy. Therefore, my strongest belief is that the best way to make a clear distinction between two children who seem to have the same problem is to watch them during their sessions over a long period of time (more than a year). This is actually one of the major claims of the book. Some initial classification is of course necessary before one embarks on treatment, but it is not usually the diagnosis itself (based on a child's initial impairments or abilities) that clarifies things in the vast category of pervasive developmental disorders and autism, for instance. Differences between two children appear through what arises in the course of therapy. In short, I am more interested in the careful narrative of a case than in the initial diagnosis. Besides, in my opinion, in the present state of our knowledge, a diagnosis at the beginning of a treatment is like a compass: it can give you the general direction, but it says nothing about the landscape. The same goes for statistical considerations, which are of course decisive. Yet, I contend that case studies over long periods of time are also decisive, though in a different way. One way of learning about the pathology of a child is to watch how he strives to overcome his difficulties. Another is to list what sort of therapy works (or does not work) with the child.

The qualitative changes in my patients soon led me to look out for any signs suggesting that acceptable communication might eventually develop. Such signs do seem to exist, though it is possible to misread them. In some developing situations, one can be slow to identify the potential footholds and pitfalls. At the beginning there is no way of foreseeing these. Sometimes apparent signs can be deceptive. For instance, an ability to manage symbols may not always mean that profitable contact will ever be made. The mere fact that a child may be competent or even quite skillful in using written language may be no guarantee that he will ever acquire a basic facility in language. Also, generally speaking, what is important is not so much what the child produces but rather the way she uses thought, her own and someone else's, in what she is doing. The pleasure a child takes in our exchange, her ways of coping with the unexpected or of putting it to use—these are all more promising indicators than an ability to manage written signifiers or pictures of objects. In fact, for arriving at a prognosis, the symptoms are less helpful than the constancy or inconstancy of the features one can observe. Looking at the surface of a lake ruffled by a breeze, the folds of sand at the base of a dune, wrinkles in a bed sheet, or the solidified undulations of cold lava, one may see something comparable in the rippling shapes. But the energy required to alter them varies hugely. What counts is not the configuration of a formal symptom but the ability of the child who has the symptom to change. As will be seen, some of these children devoid of all communication skills have developed very favorably. Obviously, I would not maintain that they have moved on from autism to neurosis. I take the view that they were not set immutably in their initial ways of being. Their disorders were akin to those present in autism, except that their habits of repetition and their shut-off state were not absolute. In some of the most favorable outcomes, the children have managed to return to normal schooling and have been accepted into the community, first in an educational environment, then in employment. However, even when things turn out as well as this, it should not be thought that the initial difficulties have disappeared without a trace. Sometimes these difficulties can still be detected in a later mode of speech. Or the child may retain some surprising mental attitudes that can suddenly and incongruously appear during a random encounter. Mere restoration of language and communication is not enough. There is still work to be done, at least if one wishes to avoid the risk of massive disruptions during adolescence.

Everything in this book derives from direct observation. The observation in question took place in conditions that were neither as flexible and unhampered as a natural setting nor as rigorous and constraining as those of set experiments. The consulting space in which I work is more designed than a garden, a kindergarten, or a house, but it is freer than any scientific arrangement. Also, even though I am relatively unobtrusive in my contributions to an exchange with a child, the exchanges he has are always with me. This means I am a participating observer, and that raises a question about my objectivity. However, the unchanging seminatural setting does enable me to make comparisons from one session to another. And since, in the main, we are dealing with courses of treatment that may last upwards of three years, I have plenty of scope to stand back and take stock, unlike what can often happen in more usual observational settings.

So this book is a reflective report on a particular way of dealing with children who are devoid of language. It aims to clarify their difficulties and to identify situations that may help in the treatment of these. Over time, there has been a marked evolution in the pathologies of the patients brought to me. These pathologies have gradually shifted away from problems of language and toward profound disturbances of relationships and communication. It should come as no surprise to the reader that my final chapter is a personal reflection on autism. This is a direct outcome of my clinical practice, and it has brought me to a general position on the conditions that allow a child to have access to the world of signs. My feeling is that these conditions depend on a proper relation between sensation and perception. Being present at the dawning of speech brings to mind the eternally insistent question of the roots of our humanity. I suspect that much research in the field of linguistics is motivated by just such metaphysical wondering. The scientist probably does well to beware of it but feels it none the less. On more than one occasion, the efforts of children trying to make sense have made me feel something akin to the uncanny disquiet that filled me when I first stepped inside the painted caves at Lascaux.

After finishing the book, some readers may well think that what I say about my practice is interesting but that it does not prove anything. They may find it too restricted, valid only for the particular children I am talking about and only within the framework of therapy, adding up to a mere series of interesting cases. This may be so, but equally it may not be so. The idea is that only general statements and experiments can really be called scientific, which in my view is true, but only up to a point. If I have read Popper correctly, a single fact running counter to a general law is enough to prove something. That is to say, I am not just telling stories of treatments with happy endings. I believe in the impact that case studies can make on theoretical positions. When I say "case study," I do not mean a mere report on a patient who has been seen only for an hour or so. I mean an account of a long treatment. When one studies carefully what happens in a therapeutic situation, one is faced with weird and unpredictable facts that often go against common knowledge and expectation. This is thought-provoking and demands a reconsideration of the various explanations one has at hand. My attitude is the following: I carefully note the strange facts I see and ask myself and my reader: how can that be? How can an autistic child who supposedly has no theory of mind go to a bookcase and get a book containing a drawing of a key just to make you understand that he would like to open a door that is closed? By requiring at least a serious reshaping of the "theory of mind" theory, this observation is important from a theoretical point of view, but it is also important to know if you want to be able to communicate with an autistic child. So I do believe that case studies can shed light on many theoretical debates. They show that theories should not always be taken for granted and that sometimes they are an obstacle to simple observation.

Part I

Which Children Are We Talking About?

Communication Disorders and Language Disorders: Rough Definitions

For more than fifty years, communication disorders and language disorders in children have been the focus of intense debate in the field of developmental pathology. There are two major schools of thought: on the one hand those observers who believe that the difficulties experienced by such children are caused by a disturbance of the higher neurological functions (a view deriving from a strictly mechanistic and cognitive approach) and on the other those who see language and especially communication as a process involving the whole person. In short, some take a strictly medical view, cognitive or neurocognitive, while some prefer not to exclude the psychic dimension and the light that can be shed on it by psychology and psychoanalysis.

These two camps, however, do share some common ground. Generally speaking, in the area covered by this book, all concerned with childhood pathology agree in making a distinction between disorders affecting speech and language and those that I shall discuss here as a disorder affecting communication. The latter is often described as a disorder of personality and behavior. All writers on this matter, whether they subscribe to a neurological, a pediatric, or a psychoanalytical view, make a very clear distinction between language disorders proper (also called developmental disorders of speech and language or dysphasias) and the sort of disturbance I designate here as communication disorder. Many psychoanalysts, like many cognitive scientists, reject any nosographical conflation of language disorder and communication disorder. The cognitive scientists see a fundamental difference between the neurological areas concerned by the two types of disorder; and the ways in which these areas are activated are probably not comparable, either. There is therefore no point in conflating the two types. This means that in so-called objective classifications, there is a clear dichotomy between language disorders and communication disorders. This is reflected in the classification given in the DSM-IV (ICD-10) and by the international classification of mental and behavioral disorders: though language disorders and communication disorders are grouped into a single chapter under the title "Disorders in Psychological Development," the subsection on language disorders and the subsection containing clinical entities with symptoms indicative of "communication disorders" are separated by three other subsections. Also, language disorders feature as such, whereas the type called "communication disorder" is seen as resulting from a disturbance at another level. The former are called developmental disorders of speech and language (and are classified at F80), while the latter are called pervasive developmental disorders (and are classified at F84).

Psychoanalysts also make this same radical distinction between something seen as a mode of dysphasia and the quite different perturbation that I call a disorder of communication. A psychoanalyst will see the roots of a language disorder as lying in the mechanism (which of course does not mean that it may be without psychic repercussions or that it will respond to a course of treatment consisting solely of retraining and exercises). On the other hand, a disorder of communication will be seen as deriving from a dysfunction that affects the totality of a child's personality. Here, too, any equation with dysphasia would be seen as specious, as the disorder of communication (with its side effects in language) is seen as a mere consequence, the emergence of a deeper all-embracing psychoaffective disturbance. Psychoanalysts see the disorder of language as a symptom whose interpretation must call on nosographical categories of a very different order, for instance developmental dysharmony, childhood psychosis, or autism. In psychoanalytical terms, to bundle "pure" language disorders with communication disorders is to make two mistakes at once. For one thing, it turns communication disorder into a discrete nosographical entity, rather than seeing it as a symptom of some other aspect of a pathology; for another, it implies that the importance and the status of the mechanism are comparable in the two different disorders. In conflating the two, one is adopting a modular approach more akin to certain assumptions in neuropsychology and cognitive science than to any psychoanalytical way of thinking.

Given all of the foregoing, why should one bother, it may well be asked, to bring together communication disorders and language disorders, when everyone, of whatever theoretical persuasion, is trying to keep them apart? Can a book written from such a perspective really contribute to clearer thinking about clinical evidence?

In my view, there are several arguments for bringing together these two aspects of disorders in communication. One of them is that, in linguistics, it would appear anomalous to reduce language to a mere amalgam of a lexis with syntax and semantics, incongruously ignoring communication. Over the years, contemporary linguistics has actually been engaged in uncovering the links between forms used in making the content of statements and the gestures, actions, and intonations that accompany statements. The pertinence of this observation is obvious in relation to oral communication between adults. Anybody who has undertaken the task of transcribing word for word a recording of a spoken exchange is perfectly well aware of how meager the meaning is when restricted to the mere sequence of the syllables pronounced and how full understanding necessarily requires the assistance of intonation as well as nonverbal communication such as facial expression, posture, actions, and gesturing. In real language, as spoken by real people, intonation, expression, and bodily movement all play a part in the functioning of any exchange. In any dialogue, all the indicators traditionally associated with the register of communication are drawn upon and associated with the register of verbal production. The fact that spoken exchange is a totality has a peculiar relevance for children. In the acquisition of language, there is constant interplay, of uninterrupted reciprocal effect, among nonverbal communication (expressions, eye contact, posture, gesticulation), preverbal communication (any meaningful voiced production not made of actual words: grunts, yells, sighs, and so on), and strictly verbal communication, whether segmental (phonemes and syllables) or suprasegmental (intonation, the melody of speech). It is, of course, important not to mix up these different levels. But is also important not to proceed as if they can be dissociated and treated independent of one another. They function in tandem. It may be the case that the neurological substrata and areas that govern them are different, but it is a fact that in spoken exchange they act together.

There is a similar interplay of elements in the study and treatment of pathological conditions. Though it is clear that the effects of a language disorder can often be distinguished from the effects of a communication disorder, it is also true that one will inevitably be confronted with cases where they overlap. With any case of serious disorder in a child "who can't talk," one should always feel free to wonder about the relative importance of the disordered language and the disordered communication. In that area of pathology, especially with young children (between the ages of two and four, say), where mistaken diagnoses are frequent, one must entertain the entire range of possible causes from the very outset. In some cases that come to a favorable resolution, there may be a residual communication disorder; in others, it may be the language disorder that persists. But, at the beginning, the therapist is faced with both registers and with the fact that they are acting together. This overlapping effect is far from negligible in the evolution of the child and in one's work with him. This should not come as a surprise: it is well known that children's purely verbal communication has its source as much in nonverbal communication (expressions, eye contact, smiling, posture, actions, and gestures) as in preverbal communication (babbling and lallation). Besides, in a more general way, whenever any disorder affects the development of language, its overall organization, and its appropriate usage, one can often find unobtrusive but incontrovertible evidence of what we mean when we speak of a disorder of communication.

So there is nothing very wrong in canvassing an inventory of symptoms covering the whole range of disorders from language to communication, as long as one does not restrict oneself to the classifications it provides. Such an inventory can already be found in at least one well-documented nosography, drawn up by Isabelle Rapin and Doris Allen, which is the starting point for many studies on language disorders in children. The authors' method was to give a complete rundown of what can be observed in children of school age whose speech or communication is deficient, with a view to reducing the diversity of disorders observed to certain groupings of symptoms. These are the symptoms that make for classification of different entities before the latter are divided into either disorders of language or disorders of communication. In other words, this preliminary perspective is not a medical one. Nor is it cognitive (or psychoanalytical, needless to say). It might be described as pedagogical: if there are children of school age who have trouble expressing themselves and communicating, how should they be classified?

An inventory going from language disorders to communication disorders is the outcome of a clinical focus on situations that confront teachers and professionals in child care, whether they work directly with language pathology (which is the case with speech therapists) or whether they encounter them less directly but just as clearly (which is the case with any teacher). Such an approach also presupposes a conception of verbal exchange as a single whole, in which spoken content, intonation, and the associated actions or gestures cannot be considered in isolation.

A glance at the literature on the subject shows that there are a great many books and articles that offer classifications of disorders in first-language acquisition and impairment of speech. In addition, a great many books and articles offer taxonomies of impediments to speaking and of the disorders that can affect first-language acquisition. Some of these studies have a narrow neurological focus. Others bring together aphasiological considerations and evidence derived from pychiatric treatment of severe personality disturbances in children. My first purpose here is to give an overview of this literature and the issues it has raised. I then outline what I owe to it and how my views differ from those contained in such literature.

In the classification of language disorders, several major lines of inquiry predominate. The initial distinction is made between multifarious disorders, with effects on communication and personality as well as on language, and more circumscribed disorders whose effects are restricted essentially to language. This is a fundamental difference, separating children who are basically all right but who find speaking difficult, very difficult, or utterly impossible from children who are anything but all right and who in addition find speaking difficult, very difficult, or utterly impossible. There is no comparison between their two different ways of coping and how they make you feel.

When a disorder is basically one of language, three degrees of increasing severity are recognized: language delay, dysphasia, and audimutism. Within the category of dysphasia, which is by far the most written about, it is standard to differentiate comprehension disorders from production disorders (corresponding roughly to the older dichotomy between "receptive disorder" and "expressive disorder").

By and large, when a language disorder appears to be of the circumscribed variety, the description of it is akin to what might be said in a case of aphasia in an adult. But if it is part and parcel of a farther-reaching disorder of communication and personality, it soon begins to show certain features related to autism and childhood psychosis. This can be so marked that expressions sometimes used in the literature, such as "communication disorder" and "pragmatics disorder," strike one as euphemisms. One almost has the impression that some authors deliberately shun anything resembling psychiatric or psychoanalytical terminology, as though the only conceivable way to make sense of any interpersonal disorder were to see it from a mechanistic perspective.

Disorders of Communication and Language

"Pure" Language Disorder		Communication and Language Disorder (F84)	
Good nonverbal communication. Disorder limited to language.		Disorder of nonverbal communication (facial expressions, movement, sign language). Disorder of prosody.	
Expressive Disorder (F80.1 in ICD-10)	*Receptive Disorder (F80.2 in ICD-10)*	*Childhood Psychosis*	*Autism (F84.0)*
Good comprehension. Poor production (halting speech, telegram style).	Bad identification of phonemes and words (poor comprehension). Inaccurate, rapid and ill-formed speech.	Semantic-Pragmatic syndrome (without autism). Flow of disparate speech (abrupt changes of subject) at variance with the situation. Poor syntax. Idiosyncratic or mannered vocabulary.	Autism with echolalia(direct and deferred). Flat or "forced" intonation.
Phonologic-syntactic syndrome. Lexis intact, grammatical words omitted (telegram style). Severe expressive syndrome. Production limited to two-word statements.	Verbal auditory agnosia. Very poor comprehension. Consequent inhibition of production.		Autism without echolalia and without language.
Audimutism			
Some onomatopoeic utterances at times. No repetition.			

The purpose of this table is to outline broad categories. Of necessity, it entails some simplification.

Before we look in greater detail at each of the proposed descriptions, two points should be stressed. First, no language disorder, not even the "pure" variety, is without bearing on the psyche. If you have impaired speech or an impaired understanding of what is said to you, this can disrupt not just your ability to relate to others but also any trust you may have in your own thinking. A malfunction in the speaking mechanism can destabilize the whole of inner life. And this can result either in massive inhibition or even in a degree of hyperactivity. Second, whatever nosographical distinctions one may be inclined to elaborate will be useful only insofar as they enable one to identify the features of disorder visible in each individual child. What counts is especially the particular and unpredictable characteristics that mark off each child from the category to which the rest of his or her symptomatology belongs. In fact, the best way to bring about an improvement in a child's skills is to work on the things that distinguish that child from the paradigm.

Accepted Classifications

Any diagnosis of a disorder in communication and language must derive from an observable and very evident disparity between a given child's abilities in speech and communication and the rest of his or her aptitudes (e.g., general intelligence, general motor skills, fine motor skills). With a child who shows large neurological deficiencies, to speak merely of a disorder of language and communication seems inaccurate. As concerns speech, I shall reserve the term "speech disorder" for those children who are incapable of using speech either in exchanges with others or in their dialogue with their own minds.

Most theoretical models are grounded in a distinction between, on the one hand, language disorders that result from a personality disorder (including a disorder in communication with other people) and, on the other, those that derive from a deficient neurological processing of speech (aphasiological disorder). The latter are deemed to be "purely" linguistic disorders. An example of this mode of classification is to be found in G. de Weck (Weck 1995). It is borrowed from the system of Isabelle Rapin and Doris Allen (Rapin & Allen 1983, 155–184) and is akin to that of C.-L. Gérard (Gérard 1991). It is actually based in large measure upon the earlier suggestions of J. de Ajuriaguerra and R. Diatkine (Ajuriaguerra, Diatkine, & Kalmanson 1959, 1–65). It is this shared body of opinion that I propose to discuss. For ease of presentation, I follow Rapin and Allen, though I refer to earlier classifications whenever possible.

"Purely" Linguistic Disorders

A first group is composed of those children in whom language disorder is the main cause of their difficulties. Broadly speaking, the existence of a disorder that is solely linguistic is revealed by the absence of any disorder in nonverbal communication. Gestures are appropriately used. There is nothing wrong with the child's linguistic pragmatics (requests, demonstrations of affect, pointing). Usually, the prosody is also good. This means it is the phonology that is affected, in particular in its oral dimension. There are cases in which the processing of written phonemes can actually be more accurate, in both comprehension and production; in learning to read, some dysphasic children can find in their new relation to the printed word the ability to "recover" a measure of facility in speech.

When the language disorder is circumscribed and mild, a term often used is "language delay." Terms such as "dysphasia" or "severe dysphasia" are used only when a disorder is more serious. In fact, a diagnosis of a disorder as language delay presupposes that the observer expects the child's language difficulty to solve itself. It is already obvious that the choice between language delay and dysphasia may incur converse risks: to treat a case of dysphasia misdiagnosed as language delay can lead to harmful consequences; to overtreat a slight language delay may turn a passing symptom into something worse and miscast forever a child's image in the family and the social group. "Dysphasia" denotes a disorder that, though purely linguistic, is of some seriousness. However, in some extended usages, this term can be more difficult to define accurately. Some authors apply it not just to cases of serious disorder in language but also to others in which language is totally absent. More etymologically suitable would be "childhood aphasia," but this term is avoided because of the possible confusion with adult aphasia, that is, the loss of language that has already been fully acquired, rather than a disorder in language acquisition.

Other authors use the term "dysphasia" to mean only the disorder as it affects children who have retained language. The fact that the prefix *dys-* means "bad," "defective," or "other than it should be" does suggest, of course, the partial retention of the faculty defined by the rest of the word that it heads. This is precisely its function in words like "dyslexia" and "dyspraxia." Each of these words denotes severe malfunction of a faculty, but not its complete disappearance. This view of the prefix respects the difference between it and the separate function of its twin prefix *a-*, the Greek privative, which heads those other terms that express the utter absence of the faculty in question. Thus we have, for instance, "alexia" and "apraxia." It is this terminological relation between alexia and dyslexia, as between aphasia and dysphasia, combined with the fact that there is a frequent association between dyslexia and dysphasia, as there is between alexia and aphasia, that largely accounts for the widespread use of "dysphasia" to mean disorders of speech which, though seriously impairing a child's language, do not entirely deprive her of the faculty.

This raises the problem of how to define the disorder of those children without language. There is, of course, the term "audimutism." However, early studies treated this as a very rare disorder. There was also the fact that the very word "audimutism," by virtue of its formation, suggests something too close to "deaf mute," apparently expressing a lack of auditory perception and not a neurological disorder. So the term was dropped. This left "dysphasia," which now tends to cover not just children who have some faculty of speech but also those who have none. The distinction made between the two categories is that "dysphasia" is used of the first and "profound dysphasia" of the second. Profound dysphasia more or less covers what used to be defined as audimutism. My own usage is to restrict the adjective "dysphasic" to children age three years and over who present a serious language disorder but not a complete absence of language. For those who present a complete absence of language, I keep the term "audimutism." However, many children who present with the audimutism profile also suffer from serious disorders of communication and personality, though the term "audimutism" was originally intended to describe cases of what seemed to be "pure," if massive, language disorder without any disorder of communication.

Types of Dysphasia

Within the stricter boundaries of dysphasia (in the sense of "pure" language disorders, but not loss of language), one finds in the literature two general focuses. One of them distinguishes between a disorder in production and a disorder in recognition, while the other, limited to the area of production, distinguishes between the garrulity of "receptive disorder" and the halting delivery of "expressive disorder." In fact, these two ways of seeing things coincide, since expressive disorder affects especially production, and in receptive disorder it is comprehension that is faulty. In expressive disorder, production is poor and evolves slowly toward a telegraphic style, whereas comprehension of language is good. With receptive disorder, on the other hand, the children's expression seems not to be a difficulty (they have a ready flow of speech), but their comprehension of what is said to them is poor. These two symptoms arise from a single cause: the children's recognition of phonemes is inaccurate, which impairs their comprehension; it also makes their pronunciation inaccurate and approximate, which is what gives the impression of garrulity. Metaphorically speaking, the children with receptive disorders can sing to the tune of language (its intonations, its broader contours), but they don't know the words to the song. Those with expressive disorders do know the words to the song (though these are reduced to the main syllable of the most important word), but they just cannot grasp the tune.

Expressive Disorder

In this range of disorders, Rapin and Allen make a distinction, according to the degree of severity of the disorder, between "phonologic-syntactic syndrome" and "severe expressive syndrome." Broadly speaking, the ability to produce a phoneme is twofold. At the most basic level, it entails first and foremost the capacity to make the sequence of movements required to produce the phonetic features that constitute the phoneme as an utterance. But, at a second level, since a phoneme is always part of a greater whole, it requires of a speaker the further ability to maintain its quality and its position in that whole, without trying to simplify it by way of omission or assimilation.

The classification "phonologic-syntactic syndrome" is used for those children who are able to produce most of the phonemes of their language, whose differentiation between phonological features is well established, and whose phonology disorder is essentially marked by omissions, substitutions, or assimilations. The disorder can be defined by the degree of accuracy of phonemes in context. By and large, the language produced tends to be acutely nonsyntactical (telegraphic style). These features are at times accompanied by more or less marked apraxia of the face and mouth: such children find it difficult to puff out the cheeks, blow through a straw, swallow, click the tongue or stick it out, or blow or wipe the nose, and they may speak with a hoarse voice. Some authors, notably Gisèle Gelbert (Gelbert 1998), take the view that these accompanying symptoms occur indiscriminately, in both the receptive and the expressive classifications. The effect of these symptoms is to impair the child's integration of linguistic movements. This creates the risk that nonlinguistic training (in skills such as blowing through a straw or swallowing) may actually exacerbate the lack of linkages in the chain of speech.

In addition to the phonologic-syntactic syndrome, there is severe expressive syndrome. It is, of course, more extreme. In this disorder, the movements required for production of the features of the phoneme are badly affected and the utterances of the child are usually restricted to a word or two.

Receptive Disorder

In receptive disorder, the second of the two "pure" varieties outlined by Ajuriaguerra, what is essentially lacking is the ability to identify the acoustic image corresponding to a given phoneme and to recognize a word solely by its sound contour. Children with this disorder have no difficulty in pronouncing a word: knowing the meaning of the word they want to say, the programmed articulation required to utter the corresponding signifier comes readily to them. In hearing a word spoken, however, such a child cannot identify it from its sound alone. The sound contour of a word has to be checkable against the motor program required to speak it. By deduction from the general context of talk, the child must identify both the idea that an interlocutor is trying to communicate to her and the word she would use if she were the one trying to say it. She then has to bring up the motor program required for this word and see whether the sound contour this provides matches the word just heard. So it is through this effort of imagination, working out what she would say and comparing it with what she has heard, that the child contrives to recognize the meaning of the words actually spoken to her. This procedure works only if the situation or context within which the child can start making hypothetical deductions is clear. If that is the case, she can respond without too many mistakes to the orders and requests put to her. But she can never directly identify a word on the basis of its uncontextualized phonetic contour. In the area of production, she may well be able to name objects from images (she has the ability to go from the concept to the motor program corresponding to the signifier), but in unprompted speech she will sometimes omit syntax words (determiners, auxiliaries, prepositions) for which no corresponding "concept" can be visualized. This is less the case with the morphology of words inflected from a root word: they mostly benefit from a sort of imitation effect, as though under the influence of the full lexeme pronounced just before. Often, too, after a variable length of time during which all the words of a semantic constellation (such as calf, cow, bull, bullock) are reduced to a single term ("cow," say), children affected by this syndrome gradually develop a very precise vocabulary. Bearing in mind the constraints that affect their ability to summon up the right word, the real nature of the difficulty they have is in accepting the existence of synonyms. At times, by their very effort to make every syllable of a word meaningful, they create neologisms, which always follow an identifiable logic in their construction.

When the disorder in recognition of phonemes is absolute, we have what Rapin and Allen call "verbal auditory agnosia." The deficit in phonetic decoding can have profound repercussions on production. There is less assistance from the memory of the mouth and voice movements required to say the words than in all other cases of this receptive disorder subgroup. It is not unknown that, to begin with, the difficulty of identifying the sounds of speech can completely prevent an affected child from speaking. However, these children do have good abilities to make sense both of written words and of another person's nonverbal communication (eye contact, gestures, intonation).

Broadly speaking, the linguistic deficit has a greater effect on the general psychic performance of children with receptive disorder than on those with expressive disorder. One suspects that an inability to understand what other people are saying (or a constant feeling of being rather at a loss) must have a strong destabilizing effect on the mental processes of a child.

Dysphasia in Association with Another Disorder

On the matter of those categories of disorder in which dysphasia is an associated factor, as I have said, some authors decline to speak of psychological disorder, preferring to focus on the idea of a mechanistic disorder of communication resulting directly or indirectly in a disorder of language. According to the ICD-10 classification, we are now in the category of pervasive developmental disorders occurring within the specific entity, autism (F84.0).

In accordance with the nosographical categories of Rapin and Allen, three subgroups can be identified, two of which involve autism. One of these associates the absence of language with autism and is defined by a total lack of linguistic production, even including echolalia. At moments of excitement, some stereotyped sounds (sucking noises, tongue-waggling with associated sounds) are produced. Such sounds, by virtue of their function and the circumstances of their performance, are reminiscent of Broca's profound aphasics who remain mute except for one word that they repeat indiscriminately each time they try to say something. In the early days of treatment, a therapist may even be moved to ask the child to be quiet, in the hope of inhibiting an involuntary production that might short-circuit any eventual emergence of language. The second category of this type of disorder is not associated with total absence of oral language. The child shows an ability for echolalia, at first immediate, then delayed. Taken as a whole, both of these categories manifest serious problems in the area of nonverbal communication, whether in its production or in the inter-pretation of signs indicative of intentions, expectations, and feelings. There is no smiling, no show of pleasure or pain, no eye contact, no symbolic play with anyone else. The child habitually locks himself into an orga-nized, self-contained, and repetitive activity that enables him to avoid relating. On the other hand, among such a child's cognitive abilities, eye-sight is particularly efficacious. Children with features of autism are well known for their ability to assemble puzzles and to differentiate between objects with close similarities, such as keys. Actually, with such children, this cognitive skill is more evident in the differentiation between objects, as well as in the association of exactly identical images (two photographs, for example), than in sorting things that, though similar, do not match in every respect. In the area of fine motor skills, these children's abilities may even enable them to write out, copy, or read words whose meaning is occasionally apparent to them (hyperlexia). Unlike what is observed in the aphasiological area of dysphasia, reading and writing skills remain fragmentary. Whether they could be of any assistance at all in the child's communication with adults can often remain a matter of conjecture.

In this pathological area, when speech makes its appearance, it turns up first as a form of echolalia, then turns into delayed echolalia, with the repetition of fragments of recorded speech or advertising jingles, for in-stance. Inversion of the order of pronouns is common, and prosody is usually poor (toneless, repetitive, or directly copied from the overheard voice of an adult model).

Alongside the children who present full-blown autism, there are often others who can show more or less apparent autistic features. These features are marked by what authors in the field of psychoanalysis call "dismantling," a process known to cognitive science as "dissociation." This is a propensity to isolate each faculty engaged in a procedure and to construct out of a minute event a whole ritual of stabilization and self-confinement. A similar phenomenon arises in the area of speech, particularly with children who make mouth noises. For them, speech is often a mode of self-referential sensuality. In the child's production of signifiers, the point is not to make sense or to engage in communication; it is rather to enjoy the sensual pleasure of moving the tongue, the mouth, and the lips.

Moving on to the area of childhood psychosis, we have another of the "associated disorders": the semantic-pragmatic syndrome without autism. This type of disorder is easily confused with the mode of dysphasia found in the child with echolalic autism. In both cases, the language produced can be relatively structured, rich, and fluent. But it bears little or no relation to anything resembling exchange or communication. This is sometimes apparent even in the intonation. But it is especially evident in the sudden jumps in the discourse of a child who without rhyme or reason blurts out statements quite unconnected to anything being said. What Freud calls the primary process of thought, the fantasizing of desires, fears, and phobias, precludes any other expression. The language uttered is a verbalizing of the inner flow of consciousness, without the slightest attention being given to any sense that an interlocutor might make of it. In such situations, the child's discourse is a reaction to the imaginary plight she is coping with, a stabilization of it, or an extrapolation from it. An adult faced with such a child, whose words clearly have a meaning, though it is a meaning that is barely comprehensible, feels ill at ease and uncomfortable. From a psychoanalytical perspective, the distortions of language are of course linked to a loss of a sense of reality, or rather to the fact that speech expressive of a fantasy world has replaced speech functioning in the real world as part of an exchange with another person. Unless this fact is borne in mind, no sense can be made of what is said. It is for this reason that the term "childhood psychosis" seems perfectly apt. Both Ajuriaguerra and René Diatkine clearly identified this category. However, a dysfunction in a child's interpretation of someone's intentions can make his disorder look more like autism, or, conversely, if he has difficulty in identifying the sound contour of words (as in receptive disorder), this can skew a diagnosis toward "pure" receptive disorder (the psychic disorder being seen as a consequence of the language disorder). In choosing between a disorder suspected to be of the echolalic autism variety and one that looks more like a case of childhood psychosis, the diagnostician's dilemma can be acute, especially since one of the further outcomes of autism can be that it takes on an appearance of childhood psychosis. For it is a fact that the latter goes on being perceptible in interactions as well as in cognitive strategies. Autistic children's interactions are poorer than those of psychotic children. In particular, they have different ways of dropping out of an exchange. The autistic child's way is to try to take refuge in some stereotyped motor activity that shuts out the adult and seems to have no relation to a fantasy world. Nothing appears to be important other than the sensual pleasure taken in handling things. This sole focus on the innerness of felt sensations closes off any possible representation in the domain of the communicable. But, when confronted with a psychotic child, an observant adult will often be able to make some sense of what is going on, even when the child's discourse becomes suddenly "out of sync." Words spoken without apparent link to the exchange soon come to sound like a way of soothing the emotional disturbance brought about by the exchange itself. The difference between the two sorts of children is no less marked in their dealings with the outside world. The autistic child carries out meticulous explorations, mechanical and fragmentary, as well as engaging in differentiations, whereas the psychotic child throws together whatever his fantasies require. The games he plays are always visibly peopled by human dramas, even when these concern dismemberment, prehistoric violence, or being eaten.

The category of childhood psychosis, and the symptomatology that accompanies it, provoke lively disagreements and differences of nosographical opinion. The fact is that the way such children present is anything but straightforward. We are dealing with children who speak, whose symptomatology lacks some of the most definitive markers of autism, yet whose relation to reality, like their speech, is sometimes strange and difficult to make sense of. There are some neuropsychologists who see a similarity between these disorders and the pathology observable in adult patients with brain disorders located in the frontal lobes (particularly in connection with the relative incoherence of things said). A second school of thought takes the view that the disorder of these children is actually an attenuated form of autism, that they are comparable to high-functioning children with autism (for instance, those with Asperger's syndrome). As will become apparent, however, in Part III of this book, in particular in the chapters devoted to Lanny, Louis, and Simon, neither of these definitions of the problem is fully satisfactory, given that all such children also present serious disorders of communication. In addition, they show no sign of the classic criteria of autism (obsessive and stereotyped behaviors or the evasive eye contact), which are found across the whole spectrum of autistic behaviors, including those of high-functioning children. In adults, the term "psychosis" denotes a measure of instability in differentiating between inner representations and external reality. Many children in the category of "childhood psychosis," though they show no signs of organized delirium, do have great difficulty in seeing a difference between effects of their own psyche (what they wish for, what they fear or believe) and what comes to them from external reality. The real difference between them and autistic children does not lie in the ability to distinguish between inner representation and external reality. A much more striking difference lies in the presence or absence of inner representations. Even though interaction with psychotic children may be difficult, one constantly senses in them the presence of relatively organized mental processes (desires, fears), whereas in interacting with some autistic children one can have the feeling that they are in thrall to their own fascination with the sensations they receive from the outside world. It feels as though they have no inner representations at all. Such a way of speaking of them is, as usual, far too cut and dried, as will be apparent in Part III, from my account of treating Charles. Here is a child who, from any nosographical perspective, is clearly autistic and yet who our exchanges have frequently shown has a mind that is perfectly capable not only of forming thoughts but even of trying to communicate them to me.

I revert for a moment to the nosographical effects of using or not using the category of "childhood psychosis." In the main, if a nosography eschews this category, it has to broaden the categories of pervasive developmental disorders and autism, which means that the concept of autism will vary depending on whether one makes use of the term "childhood psychosis." This explains the discrepancy between what is meant by "autism" in the English-speaking world and what it is taken to mean in Europe: depending on whether the symptomatology of childhood psychosis is included or excluded from the range of autisms, the meaning of the word "autism" changes considerably. And, of course, over and above the use or nonuse of a word, beyond the dividing up of a field of study, there lies an entirely different interpretation of a disorder and its nature. If the term "childhood psychosis" is ruled out, the approach taken is bound to be mechanistic. As we know, the root of the term "psyche," like the idea it expresses, goes back to the Greek word for "soul." The use of the expression "childhood psychosis" implies the assumption that a serious disorder can be essentially psychodynamic without any necessary association of it with this or that neurological or neurocognitive dysfunction. This proposition may well be debatable, but the same can be said for the practice of making too few distinctions within the category of autism. So, in this book, the children of whom I use the term "psychotic" present neither Asperger's syndrome (when appropriate, I do use this term) nor just "mild" autism.

Possible Outcomes

As a whole, the nosographical descriptions offer little by way of prognostic considerations. This is probably because of the relative difficulty of predicting the evolution of any type of dysphasia. There are, however, certain broad lines.

In the realm of essentially language disorders, probably the three most reliable predictors of some improvement lie in the degree of awkwardness affecting a child's fine motor skills in using the mouth and face; in the attention a child gives to spontaneously correcting her spoken words; and in her grasp of the written word. Generally, in children whose disorder is aphasiological in nature, recovery of the earlier language function sets in after a year of treatment. This corresponds to the period preceding the vocabulary explosion in normal children. However, the ability to diversify linguistic behavior (asking or answering questions, initiating conversation, telling a story) is more slowly acquired. Any recovery of serviceably normal language is very strongly abetted by acquisition of writing skills and the interest a child takes in these. Recovery of perfectly standard language often remains an unachievable ideal. What is important, though, is that the child recognize that his difficulties of expression must not prevent him from saying what he has to say. He must come to accept that, despite his oddities of speech, he can express himself freely.

In the category of dysphasia as an associated disorder, the most reliable predictor lies not in any strictly linguistic skills of the child but in how flexible he or she may be in the area of exchange. An ability to organize games of a certain degree of openness is an unmistakably promising sign. With a child who can allow for alternation of sequences, in which he can play all the parts one after the other, who can bear adjustments or alterations to the ritual of his session with the therapist, in other words who can show a measure of tolerance for departures from what is usual and some ability to incorporate them, one can look forward to a positive outcome. What is rather remarkable is that linguistic recovery can sometimes be most spectacular in cases where, though the seat of the disorder actually lies more in relating, the recovery of preverbal communication happens quickly (after a year of treatment) and auspiciously (without psychotic behavior or any too marked incongruity in verbal aspects of the exchange).

As can be imagined, the extent of linguistic and psychic scarring left by dysphasia is difficult to gauge. In the realm of the "pure" language disorders, the children with receptive disorder, if they have good handwriting and a generally good grasp of things written, can set about investing in reading and writing, which may help bring about their integration into schooling, as well as their gradual acquisition of standard oral abilities. Children with expressive disorders, for whom linguistic production represents a constant effort without any certainty of success, find it more difficult to put thought into words, which will always remain for them a source of emotional disturbance and anxiety. However, here as elsewhere, if children can somehow come to recognize their own strong points, this helps them to see their language disorder from a different perspective and to live with it. As for those children whose dysphasia is associated with another disorder, it is clearly rash of a therapist drawing up a final report on a course of treatment to be categorical about what relates to the linguistic disorder and what remains more generally linked to the psychic disorder.

So much for the standard nosography. I see three criticisms of the views it conveys.

Psychic Effect of Dysphasia

First, one self-evident remark: however "pure" a dysphasic disorder may be, it will invariably have some repercussion on the broader functioning of a child's psychic processes. If a child has trouble understanding what is said to her or if she cannot manage to make herself understood, it is surely unimaginable that this should have no effect on her way of being, on her feelings and thinking. In some cases, it can even lead to an inverting of the sublimatory effect of language: under normal circumstances, one speaks so as to be in touch with someone else, to circumscribe an urge and resolve it via an exchange. But if one speaks poorly, every attempt at speech brings with it anxiety about failure, which, instead of settling and satisfying the urge, merely aggravates it. In addition, when a child's production is unintelligible, or if she uses wrong words, these constant confusions will reinforce a "primary process" of thought that treats notions at the whim of passing fancy or affect, without regard for the identity of the things they correspond to. To put it another way, the functioning of the speaking mechanism always has a considerable bearing on the wider workings of the psyche and the ability to relate.

Not Two Subgroups, but Three

My second point bears on the range of causes of language disorders outlined in the standard taxonomies. As has been seen, the basic assumption is that there are two types of cause. On the one hand, there is the "pure language disorder," related to the mechanics of speech and bearing upon the production or the recognition of sounds. On the other, there is the area of relating and psychic processes, the existence of which, however, is not quite so well recognized as a causal area. This makes for one group of children who are still interested in exchange with other people, who speak poorly or seldom, but who can get by through facial expressions and gestures, and a second group whose relating to other people is massively impaired. This division is defensible, but it is insufficient, as it ignores a further dimension, the one that, for want of a better word, I call "cognitive."

This cognitive dimension is just as instrumental as the aphasiological one. But it is not, strictly speaking, linguistic. It concerns not the encoding or the decoding of the sound chain but rather the making of the bundles of meaning that precede their shaping into sound. It is understandable that, if the thoughts to be put into words remain dispersed or static, language must suffer. This is what happens when perception and action are disconnected from each other, when visual information can produce no representation that makes it possible to expect perceptions of a different order (tactile or auditory, for example), when a scene perceived remains a mere amalgam of disparate contents, or when a child cannot change the characteristic (or the point of view) that gives him a grasp of an idea or enables him to act upon it. Sometimes the disorder arises from a faculty such as eyesight or the fine motor skills, at other times from a link between such faculties.

Cognitive disorder affects not only one's relation to the world of things. There are children who have manifest difficulty in deciphering the signs that make up exchange with other people. They can see and hear what these people are doing in their presence, but the whole thing seems to have no meaning. Such children have no expectation. It is as though they do not understand, for instance, that someone who is smiling and putting on a coat is getting ready to leave. Obviously, an inability to foresee another person's actions affects all the games that deal in presence and absence: if a child cannot "see" that an adult ducking down behind an armchair is actually hiding from her, how can she ever join in and say the magic word that brings him back?

Nor is this cognitive dimension limited to the treatment of perception. It also has a vital role to play in the linkage between sensation, perception, and affect, which determines how internal bodily sensations and external perceptions are joined. The use of sign language in nonverbal communication also depends on this link. Thus, it is because the child can relate a pleasant inner feeling to the sight of a particular expression on his mother's face and to a lullaby that gives its rhythm to her facial movements that he can give meaning to the pleasant inner feeling by reproducing the lullaby or the movement perceived in her. In other words, the cognitive process that makes that linkage between inner sensation and outer perception is decisive for the construction of preverbal signifiers.

The knowledge that communication disorders, leading to language disorders, may derive from a cognitive disorder predating words can often help in the definition of certain aspects of a clinical profile. This is an area in which one works at the interface between things that involve cognition and things that are more germane to psychoanalysis.

The Function of Language in the Dysphasic Child

I have one last doubt to express about the perspectives afforded by the standard nosographies: I mean their bias in favor of the quantification of language produced, rather than an appreciation of the importance that the child herself gives to the function. In evaluating a situation, specialists mostly endeavor to count the number and measure the complexity of the forms produced, the accuracy of repeated sounds, rhythms, words, and statements, the ease with which names are found for images, or the aptness of compliance with orders given orally. All of that is, of course, perfectly valid. But none of it helps us understand how this same child uses her language. Being able to speak is not just about having a vocabulary and a grasp of grammar. It is about spontaneously using that knowledge for a psychic purpose. For the psychoanalyst, as for the specialist in linguistics, language is not made of just words. So, in order to take a true measure of a child's language, one must pay close attention to his spontaneous verbal behavior, to whatever use he makes of even the most automatic forms of politeness ("hello" or "good-bye"). One must notice how he contrives to give simple orders, whether he does it deliberately ("give," "wait," "me now"), how he speaks of objects ("it"), how he says what he wants ("no" or "again"), and how he expresses surprise ("oh," "ah," "wow"), as well as the simple observations he may make on the changing world around him ("boom," "gone"). One must also be alert to any onomatopoeias used as part of a game ("vroom vroom" or "tch tch tch"). The presence or absence of such impromptu utterances can often be an unambiguous predictor. This means that the quality of language of a child who is laboring under a great handicap is not to be gauged solely by amounts of production. It may also be measured by his ways of using what he can manage to produce. If we compare a little boy who can say "car" or "plane" when shown a toy car or airplane but who plays with them without ever saying "vroom" or "tch tch tch" and another little boy who does not say "car" or "plane" but who unprompted starts to say "vroom" or "tch tch tch" when he plays with a toy car, the more deprived is not necessarily the one with the smaller vocabulary. There are children whose speech is clumsy, yet who make the best of it, working with it, even though the forms they use may be erratic or very rudimentary. Such children are capable of eloquence with mere onomatopoeias. Then there are others whose language is technically more substantial but who are unskilled in its use, who have little to say, or who use it in strange ways. These children accompany their actions with a long and detailed commentary, rather like a bad language teacher in the first year at high school: "I take a cube. I put it on top of the other cube. I knock it off." At the same time, they are unable to ask for the book they can see on the shelf; instead, they pull your sleeve and make little noises, meaning they want you to take it down and read it. They have a command of speech when it is all but superfluous; yet, when it could be crucial, they lack it.

What is of the essence is that, however faulty the speech mechanism may be, a child must be capable of voicing both what she wants, on the basis of what she sees, and what she does not want, and of using words to make something of her representations. What is vital for the progress of treatment is for the therapist to accurately gauge the balance between the technical quality of the child's language and the role that language has for the child. Obviously, that cannot be determined unless one has been able to assess the quality of a child's nonverbal communication, the relation that has become habitual between nonverbal and verbal communication, and, if that relation is a good one, the role of any recourse to speech in the process of symbolization. Depending on a therapist's answer to each of these questions, the direction followed in treatment will vary. When the speech mechanism is extremely compromised, for instance, but there is good nonverbal communication, one's first concern will be to let the child start by making full use of what little she has left before trying to add anything to the linguistic means at her command. When, however, the communication disorder and the accompanying personality disorder are massive, and if one suspects that this is what has impaired the flow of language, one may choose to resort to uncommon or marginal linguistic skills, even before addressing other simpler and more immediate features of the case. For there are children who, though they refuse to communicate or speak, preferring to remain in their own world, will be ready to type out words on a computer keyboard if the machine tells them to. Through this device of the keyboard, one can try to establish a relationship with them, then contrive to develop this relationship through whatever shared pleasure or exchange of affect the machine lends itself to. Mind you, this may entail the constant risk that the child will become hooked on the computer, thereby reinforcing his or her alienation from genuine communication.

With any language disorder, it is not just the meagerness of the forms used that helps determine the seriousness of it. In language therapy, what counts first and foremost is to give back to speech its proper crucial role. The child must be enabled to make spontaneous use of simple signifiers so as to bring together in expression what he feels (his affect) and what he thinks (the representation that he associates with it). He must also be helped to take pleasure in speaking, in engaging in exchange, in playing with shared affect and representation through language. Clearly, neither pleasure nor play can be taught. They merely happen, by chance, without design, in the course of a session of therapy. However, if one wants a child's language to turn out as something more than a repertoire of parroted responses, if one wants it to function as a harmonious whole, then one must be ready to take advantage of unexpected opportunities.

2

Communication Disorder and Its Signs

While there is broad scientific and medical agreement about the particular symptoms that indicate a disorder of communication in a young child, there are also, as I have said, large divergences of view about how to classify the nosographical entities that they can be said to identify. For instance, no one disputes that pointing is an essential marker of good nonverbal communication or that evasion of eye contact is a bad sign, but the nosographies based upon these symptoms do not coincide. I have already touched upon the nosographical repercussions of having or not having a category of "psychosis" and how its use or nonuse alters the meaning given to terms used to define the remaining categories, in particular the ubiquitous "autism." This makes for a large problem, though that is not actually the main thing, there being two further problems of greater importance. The first of these is that certain essential features are ignored in the standard nosographical descriptions. None of these (not excluding DSM-IV) canvasses the child's history. They describe how the child presents and not what has happened to him. Yet there is a bothersome incidence of children who present with autistic features and to whom something else has happened. Many families, for example, report that their child's early development was normal and that it was not until the age of twelve or eighteen months, after an event that was relatively minor, albeit traumatic for the child (a brief separation, often caused by a stay in hospital, though for a comparatively benign purpose, or by the birth of a younger sibling) that the child started to regress and lose some of the skills that he or she had already acquired. The second thing that is curiously overlooked is the age of the child, despite the fact that the same markers observed in a

three-year-old and in a six-year-old are not indicators of the same evolution. With a child of three, optimism about an outcome is much more
warranted than with a child of six. That much is obvious, yet it is nowhere allowed for in the categories defined by the standard nosographies.
In other words, with a child under five years of age, even when the symptoms appear to justify a firm diagnosis, as soon as one undertakes treatment of the child, any notion of how the case may evolve remains fraught
with uncertainty. Any pair of three-year-olds, defined as belonging to
the same nosological category and treated by the same therapist, can
evolve in completely different directions. One of them may have to spend
his whole life in a protected and specially adapted environment; the
other, though still being a little "strange," may eventually be able to live
in the company of ordinary people. If a diagnosis is to have any value,
basically it must be that it can give an idea of how a patient's condition
may develop and suggest avenues of therapy that may help prevent the
worst from coming to pass. So we have a paradoxical situation: though
clinical signs of communication disorder appear relatively early, at about
the age of eighteen months, diagnoses do not become firm and definitive until the age of six or seven and are also unreliable as predictors. In
one way, this is a blessing, in that one can always tell oneself, when treating a child who is young enough, that the worst outcome may yet be
avoided.

All this clearly adds credibility to the hypothesis developed by a number of geneticists that it is improper to speak of autism in the singular,
that there are in fact different forms of autism. Indeed, autism is hereby
seen as more of a syndrome than a symptom. One might even go so far
as to see it as analogous to fever, which is a sure sign of illness but does
not define which one. Here, I cannot resist the pleasure of quoting the
words of Anne Philippe, a French geneticist, who has recently set forth
her arguments in favor of her present line of research into the possibility of isolating the different modes of autism. On this very question of
the heterogeneous nature of the category, this is what she says:

> Numerous studies (in the fields of anatomopathology, biochemis-
> try, functional imaging, sociocognition, genetics, etc.) have
> attempted to search for the "specific" anomaly of the autistic
> syndrome. In 30% to 50% of autistic subjects, for example, there
> is a significant increase of serotonin in the total blood supply and
> in the platelets, but this is not specific, since similar high rates of

serotonin have been found to accompany certain neurological syndromes (West's, Sturge-Weber's, the leukodystrophies, etc.) as well as hyperactivity with attention deficit. Studies in sociocognition have also sought to identify as specific certain difficulties that autistic children have with understanding of persons. Baron-Cohen, Leslie, and Frith (1985) take the view that the ability to attribute mental states to other people depends on an innate cognitive process, the aptitude of developing metarepresentations. According to this view, there is a basic dysfunction in autistic children's metarepresentational aptitude, resulting in an inability to conceive of mental relations between people and their environment and a consequent severe impairment of social behaviors. However, the hypothesis that there is a "theory of mind" deficit specific to autistic children is problematical, since there is a subgroup of such children who are capable of succeeding in tests designed along these lines.

Given that no "specific" anomaly has been demonstrated to be inseparable from the spectrum known as autism, autistic disorder is still no more than a hypothetical clinical entity.

It is possible that, with advances in investigative techniques (functional cerebral imaging, molecular cytogenetics), we may one day envisage the eventual identification of the "specific" anomaly.

Since the "specific" anomaly remains an unknown quantity, studies have attempted to categorize autistic subjects in relation to a pertinent variable (seen as a sort of "marker" of the specific anomaly) with a view to establishing whether the subgroups thus obtained presented different profiles in behavior, cognition, or evolution. Such work has included studies on IQ, macrocephaly, the presence of neurological anomalies, handedness, social interactions, the presence of hyperlexia, etc. Though this approach may well produce an operational set of categories for clinical research (giving greater homogeneity, for instance, to groups of patients studied in clinical tests), nonetheless the categorization remains sketchy compared to the complexity of the autistic syndrome.

Other studies have attempted to cope with that very complexity by analyzing numerous variables describing autistic symptoms and cognitive level in large samples of subjects by multivariate methods. To date, however, there is no consensus of opinion on the profiles produced; nor have any validatory studies been carried out. (Anne Philippe, psychiatrist and geneticist, extract from a joint research project with the author, June 2000)

So, even in the world of hard science, things are not as clear-cut as DSM-IV suggests. This is not my own humble opinion; it is the view of a real scientist, with chapter and verse in support of her claims.

In this chapter, I revisit the idea of communication disorder, focusing on the evidence used to assess the seriousness and the likely developments of any case of it. As has been seen, there are children who are devoid not only of language but also of preverbal communication, a disorder defined in the standard taxonomies as one of "communication and pragmatics." In my view, these children also show a great many of the features common to serious childhood pathologies. They show features of childhood psychosis or they present with behavioral symptoms found in autism. Such disorders are fortunately rare. Usually, these unspeaking children have adequate communication through gesture and sign language. But, if we look beyond the purely linguistic register, what is missing in them is the use of speech in that charming, amorphous, but meaningful way that one hears in the conversation of infants between ages nine and eighteen months. In addition, of course, there is the paradox of children who, though their language is relatively substantial, have strange and unstable communication. My aim here is to describe the main stumbling blocks in this type of disordered communication.

General Impressions

The most unambiguous mark of a communication disorder is the distress felt by an adult in the presence of any child suffering from it. With such a child, it is particularly hard to set up even a nonverbal exchange. The child veers from a state of apathy to one of extreme emotional agitation. She seems totally focused on existing without others and on evading them. Any slight interference by an adult, even if he intends her to take it as a sign that what she is doing makes sense for him, makes him feel like a sort of spoilsport. There are some children who make not the slightest movement. There are others who go in for little rituals whose sole purpose appears to be to calm the irksome disturbance of feeling they experience in the presence of someone else. Yet another group sets about feverish and solitary activities to the accompaniment of mouth noises and strange singsong rigmaroles. What they say is incomprehensible, except that among their vocalizations one will hear an incongruous snatch of something or other that sounds vaguely like the title of a television show, an advertising jingle, or a fragment from a story. Some of them do even more surprising things: a child who cannot clearly express a request, even by signs, will read out or spell out a written text or will be able to read off numbers without confusing 203 and 302; another one will be able to write out the name of a car or reproduce the logo of a television channel. But these things happen (it seems) at random; they sound like utterances from nowhere, fragments of enigmatic knowledge, without head or tail.

Roughly speaking, one can delineate three profiles. First, there are three-year-olds who cannot point at anything or play with an adult any games that require players to take turns, yet with whom it is possible to have, at least with the better cases, a shared interest in what they are engaged in. If one imitates the movement they make, one can generally set up a sequential alternation of repeated actions, as in the game "Simon Says." This can make them take pleasure in being imitated, then in imitating the person who has imitated them. Their games are stereotyped and self-contained, but such children are not so totally isolated inside their activity that one cannot eventually contrive to join in. Then there is a second type, composed of those who are frantically addicted to their repetitive games. They are so deeply engrossed in them that no one can find a way in. The most an adult can do is be used like an instrument or, conversely, act after the manner of an animal trainer whom the child is obliged to obey. One cannot say that such a child has no sense of other people, for if one tries to interrupt the activity or even to lend a hand, the result is immediate: the child destroys the thing under construction and, with a sudden, vehement movement, abandons the space of the interaction. With such a child, the only possible role one can play is that of a spectator: one is there as a witness and a nonparticipant. This is an exclusion that must be accepted, as must the fact that the odd moment of closeness and exchange, arising spontaneously from a child's brief mental and affective coherence, may also lead to nothing. Such instants of fruitful engagement, having cropped up unpredictably during a random session, can then peter out. The child, withdrawing into self-absorption, reverts to thwarting all attempts at cooperation. It is this alternation between unexpected exchange (why did it happen on that particular day?) and equally unforeseeable reversion to the closed world of autism that makes working with these children especially exacting. The third group is made up of children who are a little older than the others, four or five years of age. These children have a comparatively large range of spoken language, but they use it in an idio-syncratic way. They often resort to it without the slightest intention to engage in communication. In working with them, one is trying not to establish communication, which is already partly there, but to turn it into something more flexible and more diversified, something more closely approaching standard practice. Mainly, though, one is endeavoring to alter the way language is used for this communication.

The Standard Symptomatology

Broadly speaking, exchange without speech brings into play three main aptitudes: the ability to show feelings and to recognize the expression of them; the ability to use gestures and sign language to express one's wishes, expectations, and recollections; and the ability, when playing, to change roles with someone else.

In the register of affective communication, it is of course necessary to see whether a child can use signs to express her inner feelings and whether she can understand somebody else's, which may be fear, surprise, disquiet, pleasure, or nervous excitement. Over and above this initial stage of an exchange, however, one is also trying to establish whether the child can make out from the look in another person's eyes what someone else wants and is interested in. Then, if the child manages to point at something, this will mean she can engage with another mind, and exchange is almost certain to take place. In the area of role alternation, it is necessary to see whether the child can join in games requiring players to take turns, what she will do if you toss a ball to her. If she is glad to toss it back, there are grounds for assuming that she may do something similar with words, that she will be capable of taking her turn as speaker and listener. This augurs well for future dialogue. Such indications are well known, having been described in young children, notably by Jerome Bruner. They are not present in children whose communication is disordered. There are, how-ever, other things that should be taken into account, things that, though they are not tools of nonverbal communication, may help bring it about. They enable one to observe how a child stands in relation to his history, the world, and his mind. Foremost among these things is the way he remembers a previous exchange: when you meet him for the second time, it is a good sign if, for example, he is the one to pick up on some of the elements of the first meeting. What is important is not so much the fact that he remembers, but how he remembers: whether his link with the past is flexible enough to allow for variants the second time around, and especially whether his memory corresponds to a strong affect (a moment of pleasure shared, an achievement warmly praised by the adult). Another important aspect is the cognitive ability to keep an objective in mind (looking for a cube that has disappeared off the far edge of the table) while being flexible enough to adapt his strategies to the obstacles encountered. When, in addition to all this, a child can push a toy car under a chair as though it is a bridge, use a tea set to serve a teddy bear, or make a plastic crocodile bite another one, one may be sure that nonverbal communication is present and correct.

These are the essential elements. However, in order to believe that unrestricted access to language can be brought about, it is necessary to add a further condition, what I call "voicing." This condition can be satisfied if a child accompanies gesture or movement with any sort of meaningful sound. A child who utters an interrogative "aah?" or an insistent "ta!" while pointing at an object, who takes to saying "booh" when tossing a ball back to the adult, shows that speech for him is a natural accessory of action in the process of exchange and communication.

To my mind, sign language, pointing, turn-taking, and voicing mean that nonverbal communication is properly present. Memory and an ability to engage in symbolic play are valuable complements to this. If a child has mastered all these arts but has reached the age of three without speaking, then there is a strong case for therapy. The disorder that one is dealing with, however, is very unlikely to be a disorder of communication.

Residual Communication

The standard symptomatology just outlined is generally accepted and uncontroversial. The danger to be avoided, however, lies in thinking of these symptoms as a mere checklist or as a grid covering all modes of nonverbal communication. From the absence of one symptom one can very often draw conclusions that turn out to be crudely inaccurate. More important, that way of thinking will prevent an assessment of the residual communication available to the child.

Pointing

A focus on the ability to point, for instance, makes it plain that children who do not point clearly have a disorder of communication and that they have difficulty in establishing common interest with the adult. But to say, as some authors do, that these children do not point because they cannot imagine that anyone else thinks or that their own thinking could make sense to someone else is to jump to conclusions. It is insufficient to say that absence of pointing means absence of representation of another's representation. If this were so, it would be incomprehensible that when such children want to leave a room, they are perfectly capable of taking the adult's hand and putting it on the door handle that they cannot turn. Such an act presupposes that a certain mode of joint attention is established. Any child who tries to force an adult to turn a door handle must think the adult thinks and can be influenced through his thinking. The child's representation of the adult's thinking is no doubt not quite the same as it is when she just points at the handle. Nevertheless, to conclude that there is no representation of another's representation is misleading and simplistic.

Taking Turns

Much the same applies to the matter of turn-taking. Even though prima facie there may be nothing of apparent significance, working with the child can sometimes lead to a first hint of exchange. If one lets oneself be directed by the child and does nothing but replicate his actions, he can sometimes adopt, deform, and rework in his own way what one has offered. This can be enough to get things started. Not that the child's responses to the adult's advances will all be of the same kind. There will be times when he will react instantly, as though echoing what the adult has just done; at others he will wait and appear to turn aside, with a little sidelong action, as it were, a delayed echo, as though on the sly. In such cases, one is never sure that what has been produced should count as genuine turn-taking.

Sign Language

As for sign language, here too one should not consider only the outright absence of it. Needless to say, all the children being discussed have poor communication through sign language. Still, some of them do manage to show an emotional state, if only through anger or tears (and less often by laughing). It is true that signs of surprise are absent. Even so, it makes little sense to talk of an out-and-out difficulty in showing feelings. What is really at issue is the absence of surprise. But surprise is a thing apart, more complex than the other emotions. And, in any case, to show no emotion does not necessarily imply that one cannot recognize emotions in others. I remember a child with a face devoid of expression who, whenever I pretended to burst into tears, would offer me what he was holding in his hands.

Paradoxical Abilities

The fact is that children with communication disorders quite often have residual abilities that do not fit the stereotypes of our implicit theories. The obvious danger is that one may overlook such unexpected aptitudes, which must be understood if we are ever to grasp the nature of a disorder and deal properly with the child affected by it. In my view, a child with disordered communication can show in many different ways that she takes account of somebody else's thinking. Her way of showing this is atypical, not what one might expect, and the quality of the exchange is subject to variation. But it is these very variations that must not be passed over. During a single session, it is essential to note the modulations in the meaning of a behavior as well as the possible causes of them. Sometimes a tiny alteration in the setting can be enough to make the difference between a session that is successful and one that is a dismal failure; it is a clinical imperative that the design of physical contexts remain unchanged. It is less important to know what a child does or does not do than it is to observe how, and in what conditions, she does it. With this in mind, one must of course give meaning to whatever she produces unprompted, her actions, her postures, her speechlike sounds. The odder they sound, the more one should do this. It is only by the exercise of such sensitivity to minute variations that one will be able to take advantage of the instants when something in the child can be changed.

Variability of Meaning in a Sign

The fact is that, when a child is playing in the presence of an adult, the meaning of the actions he makes is not constant. Nor is it always clear.

For instance, there are actions whose communicative value is ambiguous, for the simple reason that they are the reiterated and more or less deliberate accompaniment to thinking addressed to nobody else, and communication assumes the existence of an addressee. This sort of movement can be found in normal children, too. Piaget notes an example in an act of his daughter's: the child was trying to get at a ring closed inside a matchbox; in her inability to open the box, she opened, then closed her mouth, as though in an inadvertent metaphorical transposition of her intent (Piaget 1959). So here was a movement linked to thought and not directed toward anyone else. Such a metaphorical conversion via one's own body cannot, strictly speaking, qualify as a sign. But it requires very little for it to become one, as in the following example, where a child's recourse to projection onto her own body can be seen as a fully fledged sign. She was a little girl of about fifteen months, whose father was trying to make her put names to drawings on the double page of a picture book. To help with concentration and mental focus, he folded one of the pages behind the other, then put his hand over one of the two figures still visible, so that the child could see only the one at the top. She looked at the book, then at her father. When she was sure he was paying attention to her, she put her hand over her eye. Then, with her other hand, she removed the covering hand from her eye, a clear indication that she wanted him to let her see the picture he was hiding at the bottom of the page. In this example, the child resorted to the same sign principle as Piaget's daughter; in both cases, a child made a metaphorical conversion via her own body. However, in the second case, by being intended for another person, the process has taken on full semiotic value. The action is no longer just an accompaniment to a private mental event. Working with children whose communication is disordered, one very frequently has to deal with a situation somewhere between the scene in Piaget and the one with the picture book.

The quality of a sign, therefore, is determined by the role of the addressee in the intention of the one making the sign. It is also determined by its degree of stereotypy. There more a sign is stereotyped, the less meaning it has. Take the example of a little boy of four who can neither speak nor point. Every time he arrives in my consulting room, he dashes to the board and writes the name of a French television channel, "TF1" or "F2," all over it with a marker. This is his way of retaking possession of the space and resolving the tension he feels at being left alone with an adult behind closed doors. It is also an act that has meaning but that is not yet a sign. His scrawlings say something about his interest in television, his writing ability, the pleasure he takes in showing how he can manipulate the culture of the community into which he has been born. However, it is difficult to ascribe a definite status to the writing on the board; there is no real exchange, since it is not meant for me. All I am is a witness to it. Also, it seems to be repeated without a particular purpose. Mere repetition is not enough to turn a sign into a stereotype: shaking our heads to mean "No," though we always shake them in the same way, remains a sign. The determining factor is the lack of intention. The child in question does not "mean" to tell me anything; the act is just a stage in his ritual. Even so, his writing is not meaningless. Repetition and the lack of an intended addressee do not of themselves deprive a sign of meaning. The meaning just becomes diffuse.

Dissociation of Signs

Ordinary children use a whole range of nonverbal signs: facial expressions that show affects; actions that show a desire (raising the arms, so as to be lifted up); social rituals (waving good-bye); pointing; and games of pretense or make-believe. Whatever its original category, however, each of these nonverbal signs very soon becomes detached from it and lies latent at the intersection of several different intentions. For instance, a toddler who points at a toy car that he has just pushed toward an adult is manifesting a lot of things: he shows that he wants it to be pushed back to him and is expressing a request that this desire be satisfied. But, in addition, he is signifying his enjoyment of the exchange with the adult, since the pointing of a finger is also part of turn-taking games. Furthermore, as he makes his gesture, he is aware of lacking something: the little car that he can see in front of him but cannot reach. So the pointing finger helps him to understand himself. In children with autistic traits, on the other hand, the different registers of intentionality are always dissociated. At most, one sign may be used as part of a game played within the confines of their own minds, and another may be addressed to someone else. But it is always one or the other, never both of them at once. So one may see them on the one hand making very demanding, very imperative gestures at someone else and on the other engaging in solitary mime, oblivious to everybody. But the registers do not overlap. Obviously, in the presence of an adult, when a child is playing, even if she is playing by herself, holding a toy telephone to her ear, perhaps, and pretending to listen to it, she is not entirely alone. Doing something in the presence of someone else is itself a way of establishing a mode of relationship. But the link thus made is tenuous. The therapist must have the knack of helping the child's spontaneous play to evolve without making her withdraw into herself or become agitated. As each opportunity arises, one must gently encroach a tiny bit, with the aim of negotiating a slight adjustment in the condition of witness that one has been allotted. And if the child eventually hands you the receiver, with the familiar gesture of someone telling you a caller wishes to speak to you, then you have won. Something that used to be a sign of solitary play in someone else's presence has started to become part of an incontrovertible register of exchange.

When a Game of Make-believe Turns into an Exchange

If one compares the action of a child who is pretending to telephone and the gesture of a child who is able to point, a number of differences remain. For one thing, in the early stages of the telephone game, the child is doing nothing to bring about an exchange. She is just playing by herself in the presence of the adult, without envisaging anything in particular. It is the adult who, by looking, transforms the child's hand movements into an intended act of meaning and enables him to use it as a theme to structure later interactions. It is clear that something changes when the child offers the receiver to the adult. But the difference between that and pointing remains: a child who points at an object is not asking for any sort of hand movement in response. What she is doing is asking for that object to become a focus of speech. The child who offers you a telephone also expects a response from you, but a response in the form of an action, not in the form of a commentary. That is to say, the child's assumption of thought in another person depends on an immediate confirmation through action of that person's interest: the adult must take the receiver and hold it to his ear. Also, the adult's response must be foreseeable by the child and able to be directly incorporated into her telephone sequence. In fact, the adult has to be content to repeat what the child has just done or to vary it, say, by adding at most a slight nod of the head, as though responding positively to words spoken by someone invisible. But the margins of the variable and the unexpected are small.

The Quality of Spontaneous Play

A child alone with an adult starts to play as a way of resolving the constraint and emotional disturbance that he feels. He may choose to roll plasticine into little balls or set cubes on top of one another; he may just move his fingers around and stare at them, rather than touch any of the things one has laid out in front of him; or he may even drop one of the plates of a tea set to see it bounce on the floor and listen to the noise it makes. Whatever he chooses to do, what these acts have in common is that they all defy the slightest interpretation, rule out any possible imaginative sequel, prevent any story from developing. What these acts are about is the child's vehemence. Some of these children put all of their feeling of constraint and disturbance into this motor activity; others remain detached enough to make what they are doing into something of a recreation.

With many such children engrossed in some highly compulsive activity, the scenario they develop is practically unchangeable. The most one can expect is to be used as a mere tool that enables the child to overcome some random setback arising in the enactment of the cycle and then to return to the same identical repetitions. These repetitions may amount to nothing more than dropping an object, then picking it up, or they may be a more elaborate procedure, such as running a toy car along a road between houses and into a garage. The important indicator is the urgency that impels the child's completion of the cycle. In other words, what counts is not the greater or lesser complexity of the procedure but the vehemence of the child's absorption in it. The less engrossed the child is in the activity, that is, the more the latter functions in detachment from the child, the more it offers scope for somebody else to influence it. Not that this means one must contrive to bring the repetitions to an end, but rather that, if one can engage in the scenario, if one can repeat it and then surreptitiously amend it and enrich it, and if the child will accept the variations introduced, then a space for play may have been created.

What Is a Changeable Scenario?

A readiness to accept variation is something decisive. One can be misled by the apparent richness of a child's spontaneous playing or by the way she adapts an earlier exchange and not notice how closed her scenarios really are. There are children who seem to accept and incorporate the adult's suggestions, though these remain in fact extraneous to the play procedure. I remember a boy who was making a toy soldier ride on the back of a horse. Eventually, he agreed to halt the horse at a barrier that I put in its way. But then, as soon as I lifted the barrier, he made his horse canter on as before. I thought for a time that this was a game of meaning for both of us, an interaction between us. Yet the variation was never really incorporated. The brief pause that I had been interposing had just turned into a sort of conditional reflex. All I had done, in a slightly sophisticated way, was train him to wait until the barrier was removed, so as to carry on with the cycle of his repetition.

A child's being so shut off is one obstacle, but it is not the only one. In some children, it is the opposite that prevents exchange: any contribution by the adult, however minute, results in total fragmentation of the child's procedure. She will stop what she was engaged in and either sit there in brief bemusement or else plunge into an entirely different activity. In such cases, no incorporation of suggested variations can happen, but for opposite reasons. The really important thing is that a child should be able both to pursue her own project and remain responsive to the world around her.

How Reliable Are Prognoses about Children's Evolution?

At the outset of a course of treatment, going on the various symptoms that I have just discussed, how valid a prognosis can one make? I recently undertook a retrospective investigation, in the hope of answering the following question: referring back to my notes on the different children who presented with autistic features and who prima facie belonged somewhere in the severe but not hopeless area situated between communication disorder and language disorder, can I, with each individual case, identify anything that might have enabled me to sort them more accurately into categories if I had been a bit smarter when I first saw them?

In the main, the answer is "no." There are, of course, children who do not speak and who one is sure have neither autistic features nor a disorder of communication. At the other end of the spectrum, there are those who present autistic features that are so severe and so apparently intractable that one has a pretty clear idea, sad to say, that any favorable outcome will be very unlikely. Between these two extremes, however, there are some children who have a definite disorder of communication and practically no language. These are the ones whose evolution is really unpredictable. I have learned from experience that some of them will become normal and others will go on being disabled in ways that will mark them and set them apart for the rest of their lives. Since it is not nice to think that one has spent twenty years working at something without having much to show for it, I have also drawn some tentative conclusions. They may not be accurate, but I hope at least that they show I am on the right track.

First of all, two things are self-evident. The more a child gives evidence of intelligence and the more he or she has recourse to speech, the more one can look forward to a positive outcome. However, equally self-evidently, such an observation is too vague, and it is possible to be more precise. In fact, with a child who neither points nor smiles, whose eye contact is infrequent, who does not speak (and who therefore clearly has a serious problem of communication and language), any prognosis must depend on what sense one can make of the dissociation (or dismantling) of whatever faculties he possesses. Here, there are two crucial areas: vocal production and interaction. One thing that strikes me as very unpromising is the presence of oral stereotypies. If, for example, a child not only does not speak but spends the whole time making mouth noises like "lekelekeleke" and does not even react when you imitate them, it means that he is motivated solely by the pleasant sensation deriving from his own mouth and phonation apparatus and that any sound coming from another mouth is merely a way of pleasing his own ear. For him, what comes out of his mouth is not a mark of anything that might be a subject of thought for somebody else. To my mind, vocal stereotypies (much more so than stereotyped finger movements, for instance) suggest a type of dissociation with extremely detrimental effects, since the sounds made by the mouth are completely divorced from everything else and any exchange by voice is made impossible. Conversely, a child who is practically devoid of speech, yet who at least once during a session can say "Give" to his mother or to me when he wants to be allowed to play with something, seems decidedly more promising. This is true even if that is all he says. It may be thought that this too is self-evident, given that this child speaks and the other one does not. Things do not appear so simple to me. The child who says "lekelekeleke" may also be able to sing or recite jingles in which one can actually detect language, some of it even identifiable. But, in my view, even though there may at times be a fair amount of such language and though this may be encouraging, it is not as favorable a sign as the language of the child who can say only "Give." The language in the song or the jingle, even though it may have more content than "Give," is always a thing divorced from communication. It offers no guarantee that the child is experiencing it as something through which communication might happen. I would rather deal with the child who says "Give" quite intentionally than with the child who rattles off a long rigmarole apparently without rhyme or reason (I say "apparently" because in fact if one pays a bit of attention one can always discover reasons, such as that the jingle or song is often an expression of a link between the child's present situation and some former situation in which he experienced an emotion of a similar order). Apart from the clue afforded by how out-of-context a child's vocal production may be, what matters is clearly the way a child undertakes exchange. There are children who never actually interact, which puts them straight into the very difficult category. Against that, there are many children who, when the adult mimics what they are doing, eventually let themselves be drawn into a sequence of turn-taking activities: they do something, the adult imitates it, they do it again, and so on. If one can get this far, it is a huge step forward. It is in no sense a promise that this turn of events will ultimately lead to a normalizing of anything. As yet, it is no more than an alternation of something identical; and if anything genuinely promising is to come from it, the very first session has to produce what I call integrative alternation, by which I mean that the child must integrate something that originates with you into the exchange. If, for instance, a child takes a pencil and draws a line on a piece of paper and you take another pencil and draw another line just underneath hers, a game that continues like that will turn into mere identical repetition. If, however, you decide to do something different, like draw a circle at the end of the line she has drawn, and the alternation goes on like that for a moment, if she suddenly starts to draw not only the line but also the circle at the end of it, then that gives grounds for genuine hope. What has started to happen is integrative alternation, betokening a measure of ability in the child to be in tune with someone else. In this, on a smaller scale, there is something of the changeable scenario described earlier.

Everything I am saying here is of course informed by my own "explanation" of autistic features: I do suspect that children who present such features are often afflicted by a dissociation or dismantling of their various faculties (about which I will have more to say in my final chapters).

I give here a glimpse of what I have in mind: the thing that seems to me to be most characteristic of children with a communication disorder is the way their different abilities function in isolation from each other. This can be seen, for instance, in their facial expressions, where smiling and looking are quite separate activities: either they smile or they look at you, but they cannot manage to look at you as they smile. Should they ever chance to do so, they would be incapable of accompanying the actions with any vocal utterance. It is as though each of these different skills were functioning on its own account. To my mind, the most serious of these states can be seen when this separating process cuts off sound production from the rest of the expressions, gestures, and actions normally drawn upon in exchange and communication. This tendency toward dissociation can be seen also in the area of the child's response to others. As is well known, there is a lack of congruity between the production of autistic children and what is being said to them by others. Which is why I see it as a good sign when a child is able to incorporate something originating from me into his or her activity. I see it as an indication that the child has the ability to adapt to his own purposes something done by me, building it into what he produces spontaneously. So, in focusing on these two areas, I am paying attention to whatever remains of the link between oral production and communication and whatever remains of the link to another person, which D. Stern calls "attunement." If something has managed to prevail in both of these areas, even though the broader picture may be very serious, my feeling is that there are grounds for optimism, albeit cautious.

3

Engagement with Language

The style and quality of any individual's speech depend on what the individual wants to do with it. One's relation to the spoken word, how much of oneself one puts into the sounds of language, is not the same in insulting someone as it is in making a mathematical demonstration. We each have a range of ways of speaking, our parlances, so to speak. Each of them corresponds to a usage, a need, a situation, and a particular linguistic energy, if not to a separate neurological path. When trying to establish a therapeutic exchange with a child, one must obviously work with the parlances that he or she possesses. But it is essential to recognize that, if these parlances remain a mere set of isolated abilities, unconnected to one another, if the child cannot blend them or change from one situation to another without changing from one mode of expression to another, then language cannot grow together as a whole. In this chapter, I propose to discuss this diversity of parlances, first as it develops in normal children, which will enable an assessment of what happens with the child whose communication is disordered. It will be seen that, in the range of these parlances, two major distinctions can be made: one between automatic speech and intentional speech, and another between self-directed speech and talking to other people.

Automatic Speech and Intentional Speech

In the neuropsychology of language, there is a standard distinction between two modes of oral expression: speech that is automatic and speech that is intentional. Each of these corresponds to a circuit, but also to a distinct way of engaging in the speech act. Between the two, there are differences in starting up, in delivery, and in psychic effect.

Automatic speech is an unmediated blurting out of words that can surprise the speaker. It takes the form of exclamations, cursing, commanding, or sharp warnings. Voicing the words releases the psychic tension caused by the situation. On the other hand, intentional speech (such as that used to make a difficult point in a philosophical discussion) represents a deliberate effort to put something into words. In such speech, thinking, however unformed it may be, always precedes the expression of it. The words spoken are not just a product of a situation; they give body to an idea in forms of expression that the speaker can constantly redevelop or paraphrase at will.

In both modes, the relation between thought and utterance is different, as is the mode of engagement with language. With automatic speech, a subject is freed from an irksome tension (sensation or affect) by discharging the words, whereas through intentional speech, thought can be developed.

Self-directed Speech and Talking to Others

The quality of speech varies, therefore, depending on whether it is intentional or automatic. But there is a further difference: depending on whether one is talking to oneself or to others, one does not speak in the same way. Delivery, intensity, and accuracy of articulation all vary. So does the purpose of such speech: self-directed speech is a way of experiencing one's own permanence, while talking to others is a way of maintaining a link with someone whose otherness one has first had to acknowledge. Speech being both motor process and directed communication, it oscillates between two qualities. Experienced as an activity, it assures anyone engaging in it of his or her psychic continuity through time. Experienced as an act of outreach toward someone else, it is a guarantee of contact with that person.

Diversity of Meanings

It does not follow from this, though, that any given mode of speech has an absolute meaning. Repetition is a good example. In one sense, mere

repetition of the sounds spoken by somebody may be a first way of negotiating a link with that person. This can be observed in the earliest
turn-taking play between mother and child: imitating the same sounds
constitutes an exchange scenario. The child takes his place and his part
in the game. This vocalized exchange can often replace or reinforce repetitions of facial expressions and gestures. However, when repetition is
mere echolalia, as in autistic children, for instance, the meaning is different. The repetitions, by not being addressed to anyone, constitute no more
than a game that the child plays by himself. And there are other repetitions, whispered or murmured without intonation, that represent an effort to understand what another person may have said, to find a meaning
in someone's words by internally replicating the movements required to
utter them. Here, too, repetition is self-directed speech, a mode of medi-
tative and private speech, though its purpose is in fact entirely focused
on the acknowledgment of somebody else, whose thought has to be seen
and grasped.

The Strangeness Effect

When words are spoken in the presence of someone else but not addressed
to that person, there is an effect of strangeness that quickly becomes disturbing. We are never quite sure what to think about people who talk to
themselves in the company of others, because what they say sounds as
though it were not intended to be overheard. Such speech soon becomes
a sort of noise, disconnected and extraneous to any exchange with others, to the present situation, to accepted norms of what constitutes proper,
comprehensible usage. At times, if one is to see any meaning as communication in what is said, one must resort to interpretation. I shall try to
define the nature of this untoward speech and show how a return to ordinary exchange is still possible.

Speech as Mouth Noise

There are different modes of self-directed speech. One can just make a
noise with the mouth, without the slightest thought that it might have
substance or meaning (Boubli 1995, Boubli-Elbez 1995, Boubli & Pinol-
Douriez 1997). This is what is done by children whose sole use of voice

is to utter repetitive sounds, like "lekelekeleke"or "takatakataka." The only thing that matters to the child is the self-generated pleasure afforded by the movements of mouth and pharynx. Such behavior is reminiscent of the single repeated word spoken by adults with profound aphasia: whatever the patient tries to say, he or she manages only to utter a single word, the same one every time. Mouth noises made by children, which are more like simple sucking sounds or clicking with the tongue, function rather like the repeated word, although any intention of making sense tends to disappear. Nor do these sounds reproduce the phonemes of the language. The child's pleasure in moving the mouth overrides any possible attention to phonetic accuracy, just as it abolishes anything approaching normal usage or meaning. The noise made by the mouth activity is a mere residue of the movement and not a sign that could represent a thought or a feeling.

Meaning, but Not "a" Meaning

This way of experiencing language is not restricted to children with a communication disorder; it exists in the usage of us all. It is what we find pleasurable in the apparently unmeaning rigmaroles in nursery rhymes and fairy stories. Is there any meaning in *titi carabi compère guilleri* or *pin pon d'or?*[1] Possibly not, other than the pleasure we get from repeating the jingle. However, that pleasure of speech is always subject to adherence to a text. There is a great difference between *hickory dickory dock* and the "aberrant" linguistic productions of the children I have just mentioned. For *hickory dickory dock* is an ear-catching phonological sequence that lends itself readily to repetition as a mysterious incantation or part of a ritual utterance. Once a rigmarole prescribes a set of phonemes to be spoken, what is uttered is no longer a mere mouth noise or the repeated word of the profound aphasics. Just like "abracadabra," it becomes a signifier full of an undivulged meaning, a signifier soon to be matched with a signified. The fact is, too, that one can turn a child's gibberish into a magic formula: if the mouth noise can develop and include different sounds, if "lekelekeleke" is replaced by "cracovidulo,"[2] then something can start to

---

1. A rough English equivalent for these jingles might be "hickory dickory dock."
2. *Cracovidulo*, though meaningless as a sequence of syllables, is made up of French-sounding phonemes that almost make sense.

happen. The therapist's task is then to give proper acknowledgment of the relative normalization of the phonemes and the signifying potential that it brings. For this purpose, there is a variety of means, such as astonishment: "Cracovidulo? Is that so?" This is a way of saying: "I hear what you're saying to me, but I don't quite speak your language. You have a thought there, but I can't quite grasp it." Dialogue can then develop out of the misunderstanding; and that may help the child to forgo the pleasure of the mouth movement in favor of the pleasure of shared affect. Clearly, a danger to be avoided here is to overdo it and thereby shut the child into a nonexistent language.

Speech as a Way of Existing

There are other lallations that are not to be explained solely by pleasure in the mouth. They consist of a sort of shapeless and incomprehensible utterance, a murmur that the child keeps making as she goes about her activities. It sounds as though she is making her vocal cords vibrate to convince herself that she is still thinking. In this lies another of the most ordinary sources of the urge to speak: speaking so as to have the feeling of thinking nonstop. This mode of speech appears whenever a child wishes to lend support to her process of representation, for instance when she is acting out a scene by moving toy figures, commenting on one of her drawings, even though she may be doing this only for her own benefit and though the adult may not make any sense of it, or attempting a demanding manual operation, like inserting something inside something else or a delicate construction. There is nothing to be understood in her sounds, but that is not what matters. What assures her of the continuity of her own thinking is the making of sounds, not the sounds made. In experiencing this continuity, she experiences herself thinking. In its most thorough-going form, once her language has returned to comprehensibility, this mode of expression becomes a running commentary, a sort of spontaneous stream of consciousness that, to my ears at least, brings to mind a literary association, the character in the story *Le Bavard* by René-Louis Des Forets who talks so as to keep his fear of death away.[3] This character's speech, like the child's, is a cover, designed to settle an emotional disturbance. It is neither meant for anyone nor exchanged with anyone. In her

---

3. *Bavard* = "talkative"; *Le Bavard* = "The Talker."

monologue, the child may borrow rhythms and modulations picked up from adult speech, as though trying to murmur to herself soothing words she has overheard. Her words are still intended for herself, but the music of them is a repetition of somebody else's words. We may hear this same tone in some of the children who have learned to read before they can speak: as they run their finger along the lines printed under the illustrations in a picture book, they speak comfortingly to themselves, echoing the inflexions of whoever read the book to them. Usually, this mode of speech evolves with time. However, with a child in difficulty, there are moments when speaking becomes static and remains, as it were, outside the scope of communication. The following detailed example shows how such a mode of speech differs from the play monologue of an ordinary child.

The Case of Paul

When Paul's parents first brought him to see me, he was four. They were worried about his speaking ability and his lack of interaction with others. But the views of different preschool teachers and specialists showed marked disagreements with each other: some of them stressed the fact that Paul could speak, which was true, and took the view that he would probably end up communicating like everybody else, whereas others expressed misgivings about his strange and erratic ways of expressing himself.

Paul's difficulties struck even some of my colleagues in child psychiatry as being severe enough to warrant a diagnosis of Asperger's syndrome, albeit relatively mild. As we know, autism of this kind does not compromise the intellectual abilities of a subject, who is also able to engage in some social exchange. Children with this syndrome often show little in the way of facial expression (the comparison with a deadpan comedian like Buster Keaton is irresistible), rather marked avoidance of eye contact, little reaction to the use of their own name, and relatively stereotyped requests and interests. There was no doubt whatsoever that Paul did present these symptoms. Nonetheless, what interests me on first meeting such a child is what he will do as an individual, once he becomes involved with me in a session of therapeutic work.

When he came into my consulting room, Paul went straight to the play box and started taking things out of it. It contains little rag dolls and dolls' furniture. He took the bed and laid out on it all the dolls he could find, which amounted to five people on a bed. Next, he took out the table and started to set out the chairs around it. There was a brief hesitation: one of the chairs had lost a leg, which he found perplexing and bothersome. Soon, though, he decided to lay it on the other two. Then he took up the father and the mother and the three children and laid them in a tiny bed. As he busied himself with all this activity, I could hear him mumbling things to himself in a low, rapid, and barely audible voice. When he set a chair beside the table, I thought I could make out something that sounded like "Put chair," but I could not be sure whether he had really said it or whether I had just read those sounds into his murmurings. As there were so many sleepers in one bed, I suggested that he build some other bedrooms. He immediately took a little baby, put it into a tiny cradle, and made a new room for it, saying, "Another bedroom." I was struck by his way of accepting and using my suggestions, not having expected that he would adopt that one so readily. I was equally impressed by the words he used in making the comparison with what was already there: "*Another* bedroom." His playing was rich, diversified, and capable of evolving, as was his language. Yet he was anxious to keep me at a distance. When he accepted my suggestions, it was in a tangential way, as though by osmosis, and without ever addressing me. His speech went on being the same running monologue, a way of containing his feelings by putting into words the sights and things that caused them. Paul was telling stories to himself and playing by himself: even though he was open to my suggestions for variation, there was no exchange between us.

There came a moment when Paul was in a spot: he was trying to hook two hurdles together but could not manage to do it, which made me wonder how he would go about getting me to lend a hand. His solution was the simplest possible: without so much as a glance at me, he just placed the hurdles in my hands and, by way of explanation, said, "Help me." Despite the lack of eye contact, I was pleasantly surprised by being spoken to. His mother told me it was his older siblings who had been so irritated by his habit of using gestures without speech that they had taught him to put his requests into these sorts of words. Until then, when he wanted a thing to be changed in some way, he had just plunked it into someone else's hands. Words had been required of him, which was why he had built them into the settings of his requests. Basically, however, here was a child for whom speech was only about accompanying and commenting on activity. That is, it was not about addressing other people. A new use for language, going beyond this simple commentary, was soon to come out of a new situation. Paul found a tea set and started to tidy the cutlery, sorting out the knives, forks, and spoons. Suddenly, he stopped this and asked me in an interrogative voice, "Drawer?" At home, he probably tidied the cutlery into drawers, or at least that was what I suggested, setting out a few hurdles in squares, so that he could use them as drawers. He was delighted at this and took up my suggestion at once. On this occasion, unlike the difficulty with hooking up the hurdles, Paul used his very own word to initiate an exchange with me. He was not just repeating a form of speech that others had tried to have him use. This alteration was no doubt linked to the fact that the situation in which he had to express his request was more stable than the previous one: with the hurdles to be hooked together, he did not know how to speak of the difficulty, whereas with the cutlery he knew what he wanted. From the habitual scene of the household cutlery being put away in drawers after the family meal, he could visualize the missing "drawers"; since he knew the situation and the words that went with it by heart, he had no need to imagine them. This meant he was free to give all his attention to interacting, and speech came to him naturally as a way of bridging the gap between what he could see (the toy cutlery sets to be tidied away) and what he knew and lacked (those tidying places called drawers). The reason that he managed to put a word to the missing things was very likely that he had heard "drawers" at home: whenever he picked up the cutlery to tidy it, he was probably told something like, "Will you please put the knives in the drawer, Paul?" To name the thing he needed, he drew on a situation in which the object he wanted to use was named. Which means that, even in a situation where language was well established, the child still relied on words he had heard spoken.

So Paul repeated things said or else he commented on what he was doing. The really striking thing was that, in situations where speech might have served some other purpose, he was speechless. He was as unable to make a request or state a purpose as he was to express a feeling, a pleasure, or an anxiety. If need be, he resorted to actions and expressed what he wanted by tugging at people's sleeve. If a green cube was required at a particular stage of a construction, rather than speak, he would take the adult's hand and lift it up toward the shelf where the box was. Alternatively, he just repeated what he had been taught to say. In general, when a child gives a running commentary on his activity, it is often too risky to intervene. The danger is that one might break the fragile shell that the child is trying to construct through monologue. The most one can do is imitate the child's ways of speaking and slightly alter the subject of the commentary. Usually, the child focuses the commentary on what he is doing, and the adult may be able to bias it a little toward commentary on the results of the activity. When circumstances lend themselves to it, change can at times happen. I remember, for instance, a child who was totally absorbed by writing out the names of different fruits on the whiteboard. What mattered for him was the pleasure of listing things. But then he gradually came to accept the idea of drawing a banana under the written name and eventually to pretend that he was taking the banana from the board and handing it to me. So his activity had been slowly transformed. His frantic writing at the board, the essential purpose of which was to keep me at a distance, had been succeeded by something else, and we were then able to play together with imaginary fruit because we were both looking at a word. Speech, which had begun as the mere reading out of words on a board, had imperceptibly turned into a genuine exchange.

Exorcising Strangeness

To prove to yourself that you exist, you can keep up a nonstop commentary on everything you do. But you can also use words to banish the strangeness of situations that arise, perhaps by making associations. Paul, for example, was at the lunch table one day with his mother, eating a yogurt, when he asked her for sugar. When his mother passed him the salt cellar by mistake, he noticed this and immediately said, "It's the wrong foot!" Clearly this was not just one of those charming things children will say; it was also something he must have been repeating, having heard his mother say it when he put his left shoe on his right foot. How, though, are we to understand the relevance of the analogy and the surprising transposition he made? An ordinary child would have said something simpler: "That's wrong," or "No, not salt," or even "No, sugar." Paul's process was different, as though he were unable to directly put a word to his present sensation without having to detour first through the memory of the mistaken shoe. To define the feeling he had when his mother passed him the salt, he took words and images from the earlier situation. And, in coping with his untoward feelings and putting them at a distance, it was her words that he took.

Talking to Oneself to Soothe One's Affects

In talking to oneself so as to experience one's own psychic continuity, one can do as Paul does and make links with the past. This is a way of feeling continuous, despite the emotional perturbances arising from the incessant tensions of the world. Talking, even to oneself, is a way of avoiding being overwhelmed. If ordinary children are to find comfort in talking to themselves, they must have a solid link with other people and be able to draw support from the idea of an addressee for their words: they must talk to themselves in the presence of others and say things that remain sharable. A balance is then struck between talking for one's own benefit and talking for somebody else's. Talking in someone else's presence remains a way of talking for one's own benefit. But a child can allay a worry by expressing surprise, and that reaction can be strengthened by somebody else's positive reaction to it. This can be seen in the earliest meaningful interjections of young infants saying "Oh" and "Ah." Such voicing expresses emotional perturbance, but it is a perturbance that is calmed by the sharing of it that language makes possible.

Distancing through Speech

In order to balance her inner feelings, a disordered child tends to turn away, to turn off relations with other people when relating becomes too perturbing. Language becomes a forlorn vestige, without head or tail, an echo from nowhere; relating often turns into set expressions, remembered from a reading of a story, a cartoon film, the words of a song, or an advertising jingle, with no variation either in tone or in the arrangement of the words. It sounds as though the child's recourse to anomalous speech is a way of coping with the moment's affect, but in a manner that neither communicates it nor supports it by sharing. Such a child will suddenly shout, without rhyme or reason, "'No, no,' said the little red hen." Then, in a garbled and almost incomprehensible sequence, she may rattle off the rest of the story as it has probably been told to her many times over. Though such speech becomes automatic, it does not lend itself to interpretation, unlike swearing or shouts of surprise. It takes time to understand where it comes from and what it means. The exact situation from which it derives can be difficult to establish. Once this origin is identified, it is often found to be marked by an affective tonality that provides a link with what the child experiences at the moment of utterance and the earlier context in which the phrase was heard. In order to take these words from nowhere and work them into an exchange, that earlier context must of course be discovered, and whatever links remain between it and the child's affect must be put into words. This affect may be associated with the child's actual experience ("Yes, that's the book your Mama reads to you at night, and it's the one you like best, isn't it?") or with a situation from a book or a film ("Yes, and you're just like the little red hen, because you don't like it when someone tries to frighten you because you don't want to do something."). When this works, it helps to locate a link, a bond of shared feeling, between the little red hen in the story and the child's own experience in the present. More often than not, this therapeutic action on a child's speech makes the adult feel much better; but, sad though it is to say, there is no way of knowing whether the child feels much the better for it.

Speaking Too Close to the Bone

One can be taken aback by children who say things that sound too close to the bone. In my view, the saying of such things corresponds to a sensation and not to any representation associated with an affect. Here are two examples. The first concerns a child whom I was seeing for the first time, with his parents. The little boy was terrified by the whole clinical set-up and kept well away from our conversation, hiding behind an armchair. Then, as his mother was telling me how anxious she was about the coming year, he suddenly popped up and called out, "What's up, Doc?" This question, with its clear reference to me as a doctor, is at one level a request for a pronouncement on him. But it is also a reference to a cartoon, echoing what Bugs Bunny says to Elmer, his pursuer. He usually says it when Elmer is holding a gun to his head, immediately before escaping and diving into his burrow to finish off chewing a carrot with a snide glint in his eye. The boy's statement expresses all of this, too, and with such amazing aptness that it is almost unseemly: he feels pursued, targeted by my eyes, and he contrives to say as much. It is obviously not easy to grasp the role of language in his psychic process. He must be drawing on the memory of the cartoon (the visual memory of the scene, as well as the memory of words spoken) to impose some stability on what the consulting situation with me made him feel, and perhaps also to relieve himself of that distress through speaking the words spoken by the rabbit. Certainly, the purpose of his speech was not to engage in exchange or to process the psychic tension that he was experiencing but to get rid of it.

This way of giving form to irksome and overwhelming feelings so as to expel distress is quite common among children who speak in a "sidelong" manner, as it were. My coining of "sidelong" as a description of speech is merely an intuitive attempt to characterize the way of speaking peculiar to such children. By using it, I hope also to avoid the whole issue of their nosographical classification, since my focus here is on the odd way in which such children use language.

My second example concerns a little girl whose parents had brought her to keep a regular appointment with me. That morning her father had gone to fetch her so as to drive her to meet her mother at my consulting room. However, this had proved very difficult: when they got downstairs and he went to get the car, the child suddenly stood still and started shouting, "Help me! Oh, please help!" This dramatic outburst may not sound like a borrowing, but that is what it is. Though full of meaning, it is also a word-for-word recycling of a line that the little girl had often heard. It was a quotation from a scene in the Disney film *101 Dalmatians* that she was forever watching on cassette, even when she ran it through back to front. The scene is one in which the horrid Cruella DeVil has come to steal the puppies while their owners are away so that she can kill them and have them made into a coat. On the sidewalk outside the house, as the puppies are being taken away in a luxury car, Nanny, unable to prevent the kidnapping, starts to shout, "Help me! Oh, please help!"

To me, what is important here is that the child's words were both appropriate and inappropriate—inappropriate, because she was shouting in a void, not addressing her father or actually calling for help to anyone, but appropriate, too, because in this way she could relive the scene from the film and control her present terror. She was also expressing, in a particularly apt and violent way, a feeling of total helplessness at being kidnapped. How can one make sense of this lengthy detour of speech through a scene in a film? How is it that the child is unable to speak for herself but can avail herself only of a visual and auditory memory that she then reproduces word for word?

To trace this detour, it must be supposed that the situation as experienced by the child in the present (her father coming to fetch her) set off in her a violent sensation. This led to considerable distress on which the child could get no purchase. However, such an uncontrollable inner state did not result in an outburst of motor activity: she did not have a tantrum, she did not start crying, though she did not manage either to give her affect a personal mode of expression. What she felt was unrepresentable, though she did manage to correlate it with another sensation of the same type: the one that, when she was watching *101 Dalmatians*, made her feel all the helpless panic of Nanny confronted with the kidnapping of the puppies. Shouting, "Help me! Oh, please help!" was a way of internally actualizing the scene from the film, linking the present sensation with the remembered one via an association through the images and the words of the film. The present sensation could then be stabilized. In addition, shouting like Nanny presumably let the child expel and free herself at least partially from her sudden distress. By repeating what she had heard in the film, the little girl circumscribed her feeling of the moment, vented it, and got rid of it.

So there are children, such as this little girl, for whom language is not a means of communication. Why she expressed herself by quoting a line from the character of Nanny in *101 Dalmatians* rather than throw a tantrum and be dragged screaming and struggling to the car or more simply say something like "No!" or "I don't want to!" remains a mystery. It is a fact that to express refusal or put up resistance, one must have a clear representation of what one wants and does not want. Without any such representation, the sensation experienced remains more like a physical sensation, close to panic, and language cannot cope.

Sudden utterances of this sort can be upsetting for the adult. Even if one remembers the scene in *101 Dalmatians*, it can be hard to recover one's balance sufficiently to keep the dialogue going and to think of how to use "Help me! Oh, please help!" as a fruitful theme for future exchange. Such a cry of distress, though touching, often leads to nothing. The unhappiness put into the words can only be expelled by them, but no more. This is a process that may so effectively neutralize the child's tensions that his or her psychic activity return to zero. All possibility of representation is nullified: the cry disperses terror, but it leaves no thought behind.

Speech Disorder or Disorder of Thought?

The use of language by some children recalls the aberrant usages described by Freud in his article "The Unconscious" ("He's an eye-roller"; Freud

1952, 112–113). The characteristic of these usages is that the children take all sorts of liberties with signifiers, which they use without observing syntactical or lexical rules.

Usually, this discrepant usage is related to their inability to take account of contexts in choosing their words. Pascal said: "At times, Paris must be called 'Paris'; at others it must be called 'the capital of the kingdom.'" In both contexts, it is the same city, but style requires it to be different. Some usages, to be appropriate, must take account of the situations that the chosen words and expressions have to fit into. Not all children are able to manage this type of modulation. When it occurs to them to name a thing, some of them call to mind the situation in which they heard it being named, then repeat the term used, without the slightest variation. Since it is the memory of a situation that helps them find the word, they can choose no other. The fact is that, in order to manage such variations, one must be capable of putting a name to a thing without difficulty, without even having a particular context in mind; it is in that very ability to bring to mind a word severed from an image or a concrete situation that the problem lies for these children. Sometimes, if deprived of the help given by an image or a situation, they will even draw on the words being used in the current exchange or that are brought to their minds by things being said. This can suddenly sound like a disconcerting change of subject, and one finds oneself in a dialogue full of unexpected and often unfathomable twists and turns. One understands all the words, but the exchange is still hard to follow. Its style may turn poetic, a little mannered, or too exact. The following is an example of what I mean. One day I asked a child who had intermittent difficulties of this order to tell me the name of a teddy bear he had just mentioned. Actually, the teddy had no name, which in itself is quite peculiar. But what was more peculiar was the words he used in reply. My question was asked in this way: "What do you say when you call him?" To which he replied: "I name him by his common name." Those were his exact words, not "I call him Teddy" or "I say 'Bear'" or some other ordinary answer. His form of words was in no way defective; in fact, it was perfectly correct and less ambiguous than my own. Yet, it struck me as rather anomalous. It sounded like a translation of an idea originally expressed in a foreign language or like a piece of written prose that crops up in the middle of a chat. It was out of keeping with the casual familiarity of tone in the rest of our exchange. However, it is possible to discover how it came to be formulated. In trying to answer my question, the child must have remembered that a question like "What's he called?" gets answered by a "name." So what came to his mind was the word "name"; in the construction of an answer, this word was the focus around which the rest was assembled. Hence his form of words: "I name him by his name." Not having a name for his teddy, he added a general qualification to the word "name," making it into "common name." Presumably because he finds it difficult to summon up words, he found he needed to rely on the word "name" twice: first, to manage to use the verb "to name," which is directly linked to it, and, second, to make the expression "common name." But, having found the terms "to name" and "common name," he could not diverge from them. He is unable to reword things, to paraphrase his own meaning, even though he is quite aware that the words he has spoken are out of keeping with the style of the exchange. He can find a noun if he can "see" a thing or if the present exchange brings up words that prompt others to his mind. However, he lacks the flexibility to be able to rephrase what he is thinking; and this is what sometimes makes him say things that sound affected or stilted. Despite appearances, the mechanics of his speech are in part responsible for what seemed at first sight to be a disorder of communication. Something of this can be seen in a poem that he wrote about a rainy day during a session:

> C'est un jour dur à décrire,
> tant on pourrait venir en ligne de mire.
> Quand la bise fut venue,
> pas un endroit pour se cacher.
> Même pas un endroit dépourvu
> s'en viendrait à nez.
> L'averse et la tempête,
> tant en emporte la fête,
> qu'il ne reste plus qu'à souhaiter
> qu'un nouveau jour pourrait arriver.[4]

---

4. Translator's note: These ten lines, neat in rhymes, passable in grammar, and containing some striking idiosyncrasies of vocabulary, are as difficult to translate as any subtle poet's versified wordplay. Roughly, they say this: "It's a hard day to describe, / because you could come so much into line of sight. / When the north wind did blow, / nowhere to hide./ Not even a place without / would come to your nose. / Showers and storms / blows the holiday so away / that all that's left is to wish / for another day."

I do not intend to comment on the whole text, except to say that the two expressions *venir en ligne de mire* (= literally "come into line of sight") and *venir à nez* (= literally "come to nose") correspond to very precise and fixed meanings for the boy. He explained to me that *Même pas un endroit dépourvu s'en viendrait à nez* actually means *Même pas un abri qui puisse nous venir sous le nez* ("Not even a shelter that could come in front of your nose"). I add that he did not speak like this all the time and that it had been his choice to write poetry, the syntax and lexis of which are freer than those of prose. Even allowing for that, the fact is there is something intriguing in the way the meaning is put together and in the lack of concern for what anyone else might or might not understand. Obviously, in working with a child who has this sort of difficulty, one's whole aim is to bring him to a realization that abiding by syntactical and lexical rules is not a matter of indifference without having the effect of making him abandon speech and exchange altogether.

When Humpty Dumpty is convinced that he is the one who is in charge of words and can make them mean what he wants them to mean, how can he be brought to accept that that is not how things really work without making him start to wobble on his wall, then fall to the ground, breaking his fragile eggshell?

With a child like the one I have just described, the whole question of how to diagnose his disorder remains unresolved and difficult. At school, he was a child who performed brilliantly. He had friends and had little difficulty maintaining a social life, though his classmates, who at times found his stilted expressions hard to understand, did pick on him rather readily. One could easily imagine that, as an adult, he would be able to fit reasonably well into a socioprofessional world and bring up a family. Yet, the fact remains that, to this day, his ways of expressing himself are curious. It is hard to tell whether the disorder is limited to his apparatus for reasoned speech or whether there is a farther-reaching disorder of the whole way in which we engage with other people and their minds. European psychoanalysts would prefer to speak of a psychotic tendency progressing to neurosis, a form of words without equivalent in the international classification. The category the child would most closely correspond to in the international classification is Asperger's syndrome. Yet to diagnose him in accordance with that category would be to overlook the facility with which he can engage in exchange and relate to others. A slightly less blunt instrument for analyzing the evidence is required if we are to be able to think usefully about appropriate therapy.

Self-directed Speech Borrowed from Dialogue

I have just reviewed several different modes of self-directed speech. In all of them, the primary intended addressee of what is said is the speaker. There are, however, other cases in which this inner-directed language is actually the second stage of an exchange with somebody else. It has become internalized dialogue, an indirect inward-directed language, deriving from the spoken words of another person appropriated and absorbed. A striking instance of this can be seen in children without language disorder who, when they are tempted to transgress a prohibition, say "No" to themselves by way of reinforcing their shunning of disobedience. It can be seen, too, when one asks a child to comment on an image. What she says will at first sound as though she is just doing what she is told, responding to the suggestion that she should speak. Then, if she starts to become interested in the picture, she will draw on the way the question was worded, as she develops an idea that will have only a (relatively) distant relevance to the questioner. As she gradually and steadily loses the sense of urgency conveyed by the initial request, a new register of inner-directed language can emerge.

As can be seen, there is a range of diverse ways of speaking, some of which may seem strange, though in fact none of them is completely foreign to us. However, a set of ways of speaking, a set of individual parlances, does not add up to language. If language is to become a whole, stitched into the fabric of a child's feelings and thought, the different threads of these fragmentary sets must be woven together. This process is both a miracle and an everyday occurrence. But if something has hampered this process, one cannot help being taken aback by it, at least to begin with. The few ideas one may scrape together about the causes of the disorder, the knowledge that they are psychic as well as mechanical, may not take one very far. Every treatment is, in its own way, a variation on the same story: I am an adult who is trying to play a game he does not understand with a child who keeps on making signs about it. This is a practice that is both unforeseeable and paradoxical; it is now time to go on to the principles that apply to it.

Part II

Principles of Therapy

4

Joint Attention

Generally speaking, the question of what it is that prevents a child from speaking and communicating has different meanings, depending on whether it is asked by an aphasiologist, a neuropsychologist, a psychiatrist, a pediatrician, a speech therapist, a psychoanalyst, or a specialist in occupational therapy, psycholinguistics, linguistics, or education. Each of these diverse approaches gives a different meaning to the terms "speaking" and "communicating" and also to the idea of what "prevents." Notably, there are some practitioners for whom the key factor is a breakdown of the neurological mechanism, while others suspect a farther-reaching disorder that bears on a child's whole personality and ways of relating to others. There are always two ways of thinking: on the one hand, some focus on the neuron; on the other, some focus on the psychic process. The first school of thought speaks of deficiencies, the second of defense mechanisms. According to the first school, there is something missing in the child, who must therefore be coached and reeducated; the second school insists that there is nothing to be taught, and especially nothing to be asked of the child, that the way to proceed is to wait for the appearance of a spontaneous urge to communicate and the emergence of speech, however rudimentary and fragmentary these may be. Such assumptions lead to professional mindsets that are very familiar to anyone working with children in difficulty. Though I mention these fixed assumptions, I have at least two reasons for not sharing them. The first is that in any reeducative practice there is bound to be a measure of psychotherapeutic effect (by the nature of the thing, I mean, and not because the reeducator turns into a psychoanalyst). This is a point that has often been stressed by René

Diatkine. No speech therapy ever works the way a teacher of foreign languages works on "consolidating" pupils' grammar or vocabulary, nor is it reducible to a retraining of impaired motor skills in the mouth and phonation apparatus. The second reason is that the problems must be posited not in black-and-white terms but in terms of conflicting complementarity, at least as far as working with children who do not speak is concerned. With a child who does not speak, one cannot entertain notions related solely to psychic processes, any more than one can think solely in terms of neurological deficiency. One must be aware of both and be ready to work within the conflicts between them. What is difficult in this is to recognize the conflicts and not to behave as though a good dose of wishful thinking will make them disappear. The lack of language is always a consequence of a conjunction of mishaps that, though initially separate, very quickly begin to have ill effects on one another and turn into a vicious circle.

Acquisition and Learning

No one ever learns his native language; no one ever learns to communicate, either. If these skills are not acquired naturally, what can be done?

If one leaves aside straightforward learning difficulties (with arithmetic, for instance, or learning to read), so as to envisage solely the sorts of disorders that can crop up in the acquisition of a native language, then one question becomes particularly pressing: it concerns the problematical link between the neurological mechanism and the process of symbolization, the relation, that is, between the functioning of a technical ability (implying possible retraining and teaching) and some other thing that is far greater and much less definable. The fact is that what is missing in a child without language or communication cannot be taught. What you have to do is get the child to acquire it, and that is something radically different.

Roughly speaking, the difference between acquisition and learning comes down to a few pairs of simple opposites: acquisition is done in a natural setting, among familiar people, whereas learning requires a designed and unfamiliar setting with special people, also unfamiliar; acquisition happens inadvertently and through play, but learning requires the effort of paying attention and aiming at intended success. Acquisition is ecological and automatic, while being also a private thing; learning is logical and deliberate, while being also a social thing. The closer one comes to the acquisition end of the spectrum, the harder it is to distinguish the psychic process from the mechanism. Concerning the matter at hand (acquisition of communication through expression, signs, and native language), it is impossible to make any distinction between the mental impulse that makes for expression of thought or affect and the technical translation of it into action and speech. This, however, is not at all the case with expression through a second language.

The Range of Choice

The treatment of children with difficulties of communication and language is usually conducted in two or three sessions a week. In addition to this, of course, the children will also be attending either school or some other place of care, depending on their needs and abilities. There is almost total agreement on this. But any treatment must also take account of the specifics of the process of acquisition. A problem can arise when it comes to choosing a mode of treatment, since the range of available techniques is huge: psychotherapy, psychotherapy-cum-logopedics, speech therapy, small-group work, mother-child therapy, psychomotor treatment, or psychoanalytical semiotherapy. Though it can, of course, be difficult to set down in the abstract a set of determinants that govern the choice of treatment, it is possible to define a few principles. In cases where the importance of making progress and the specter of "falling behind" have been overstressed to the child and have made both the mother and the child lose the pleasure of play and exchange, mother-child therapy may be indicated. If, however, a child presents great cognitive or motor difficulties, if his way of relating to an adult constantly requires him to use great space, if the slightest impingement on his own activity brings out loud shows of exasperation, then psychomotor treatment may be called for. It can often result in more constructed and harmonious motor function, and more diversified and less crude sensational reactions, which can lead to the establishment of affect and a well-tempered experiencing of speech. If a child's excitability makes individual treatment difficult and if the presence of other children can help in the areas of self-identification and support, then small-group work may be most beneficial. Or, again, if the child has some awareness of having a disorder, shows a willingness to improve, and has good experience of socialization (through board games like *le jeu de l'oie*,[1] for instance, or school work), then the best course to follow will be speech therapy (which does not mean these are the only cases in which it will be appropriate). Then there is my own line of business, what I call psychoanalytical semiotherapy (it had to be called something). This approach appeals to me when a child's prelanguage communication is still embryonic or when there is some aberration in the use of language. It entails creating circumstances that can lead to exchange and promote the initiation of communication requiring speech.

These, then, are the principles. Some of my colleagues may well take exception to this way of presenting them, though I see my purpose as being less to issue a set of instructions for use for each of the different therapeutic methods than to put into a broader perspective the particular treatment that my own practice allows me to speak of.

Psychoanalytical Semiotherapy

A choice of therapy is not just a choice of technique. First and foremost, what one is choosing is a way of being with a child. My own way of relating is at times not very different from those favored by other therapists, such as speech therapists or psychomotor specialists. However, I should stress that it does have some peculiarities. First of all, my approach is not organized around any clearly defined plan. I do not explicitly aim to transform this relation with the child so as to foster in her any greater ability in communication or language than she already has. I tend to suspect that, if such an achievement is to take place, then it will, almost of its own accord. Adhering to a preconceived plan can be a good way of not noticing the unforeseeable hints that the child can supply. Being adventurous can lead to success. It is a fact, too, that most of the children I see have already been through the hands of other educators who are as diverse as they are qualified. The real reason that nothing has worked with them is that therapy has been based on a plan. Like the proverbial horse, they have been taken to water, but no one has been able to make them drink.

With a child who cannot speak, waiting for speech to happen can clearly be risky. I do not believe that merely sitting and waiting is appropriate under all circumstances, with every child of whatever age. The risk should

---

1. *le jeu de l'oie*: a French board game for which Chutes and Ladders is a rough cultural equivalent.

be taken only if the child is simultaneously receiving other, more directly reeducative treatments. But what is required is a space where the child can feel constantly in charge of what goes on. The only way this space can entail no disadvantages for the child is for its designer to be sure that other people are teaching what has to be taught.

Side Effects of Psychoanalytical Training

My work as a semiotherapist is in large measure influenced by my background and my having absorbed a culture of analysis. Admittedly, given that the children I treat are unable to speak and that their grasp of communication is often tenuous, any psychotherapy I might engage in is bound to be nonstandard and is quite unlike what one can do with very young children (at the age of two, for example). I make practically no interpretation, and I am convinced that in-depth psychotherapy can be conducted without interpretive accompaniment. I am quoting Winnicott, not trying to be provocative (Winnicott 1975, 86). My background in analysis has given me the habit of being closely aware of my own countertransference, that is, the feelings and sensations I experience during a session with a child, which I make a constant effort to focus on and tease out (no easy thing to do). I suspect this background has also given me my interest in play and in noting how the nature of play varies over a course of treatment with a given child. I also have recourse to analytical theory as a way of understanding children's ways of experiencing themselves and of making sense of me in our exchanges. The fund of ideas I draw on is nothing if not standard: Freud, of course, and (as is common among analysts working at the frontiers of child psychosis and autism) later related writers who have endeavored to refine our knowledge of the thinking, the affective domain, and the personality of very young children. I am referring to writers in English such as Melanie Klein, Donald Meltzer, Wilfred Bion, Frances Tustin, Esther Bick, Hanna Segal, and Donald Winnicott, as well as to others in French, like René Diatkine and Serge Lebovici (all of whom can be found in the bibliography). These authors are rich in insights on the complex process by which a human being goes about becoming individuated (or not, as the case may be). They help us understand both how human beings, through coping with their inner tensions, come to have a sense of their own autonomy and a representation of it, and also the degree of independence they can give to their love object (at least in cases where individuation is achieved in the absence of it). All these considerations obviously presuppose a pre-Oedipal perspective: the classic triangle of father, mother, and child has no immediate relevance here. With the benefit of experience, I have of course cobbled together my personal metapsychology, with which I try to understand what I see and feel. In general, the propositions that recommend themselves to me tend to be those formulated in terms of movements and processes, rather than ones based on figures, positions, and mechanisms.

Some Loss of Identity

The most singular thing in semiotherapeutic work is probably the therapist's position on the question of identity. It is not difficult to state what a semiotherapist isn't. No semiotherapist is ever a surrogate mother, for example. Even though one's role, unlike that of others who have a professional involvement with the child, such as schoolteachers or health workers, is not to instruct or to administer a remedy, one remains a stranger for the child. The feeling of complicity she has, the sense of continuity of relationship, are not as immediate as with her mother. Also, the therapist is convinced, perhaps more so than the mother, that communicating with somebody else may not be the first stage of communication. There are children who cannot communicate with other people until they can communicate with themselves. It is not easy to keep plugging away at encouraging nascent communication when one is not the addressee of it, especially if one is anxious about the other person's ability to engage in exchange.

Basically, when I work as a semiotherapist, if things are to go well, I have to feel unburdened by my own identity, out of reach of the pain of separation, divorced from the unbearable violence done to me by another's otherness and the fracturing urges (the desire to take possession, to destroy, to consume the other, to absorb the other). There is an affective contact of sorts, without clear contours. I slip out of myself; I stop being a person and become as formless as an atmosphere. One must be capable of taking a degree of pleasure in sloughing off one's individuality and working the illusion of one's own disappearance despite being still physically present. What this amounts to is a particular way of supporting someone, of being open to another's anxiety, hatred, or depersonalization, while avoiding excessive guilt feelings if one finds it all incomprehensible or is overcome by sudden boredom. It is a way of being able to put up with vagueness without becoming depressed and without understanding.

The Initial Agitation

At the beginning, most of the children I see have little scope for properly flexible play. Their anxiety and agitation are all too strong. Interestingly, during the early consultations, the therapeutic setting and the presence of the adult have the effect of stimulating the anxiety and agitation. As René Diatkine has pointed out, the experience of being alone in an office with an adult of uncertain intentions is one that a child finds worrying, odd, and exciting. There is no recipe for bringing this state of agitation to an end, or for calming one's own agitation. It may be thought that the anxiety and agitation of an experienced therapist pale into insignificance when measured against those felt by an autistic child. But anyone who has spent half an hour alone with a child who not only will not speak but systematically declines every single suggested game or exchange will appreciate the strength of the anxiety, or the state of utter helplessness, that this can induce. On the one hand, it is apparent that the child busying herself as you look on wants you to take an interest. But the simultaneous rejection of any offer or word, any encouragement or question (as well as the fact that her play is so enigmatic and repetitive), is a way of excluding the person whose interest is desired. One has to accept and put up with this ambivalent way of relating, though the temptation to suggest or ask something soon becomes all but irresistible. One eventually realizes, of course, that the only result of any such intervention is to increase the feelings of insecurity already induced in the child by adults' questionings. So a measure of educated self-discipline is required if one is to avoid jumping to conclusions about ways of dealing with the child's enigmatic procedures or dreaming up wild diagnoses, rather than just sitting there quietly and observantly, taking an interest in something that defies comprehension. This attitude is a token of an ability to cope with one's own anxiety and agitation. Without it, one could not possibly go on being interested in observing a child while having to rigorously respect her way of keeping you out of everything that she does.

The Therapist's Modes of Thought

Sitting there saying nothing and doing nothing allows time for thinking. In fact, thinking is the only thing that makes the passiveness bearable. Sometimes one's thoughts start to wander: the mind is elsewhere, full of nothing in particular, until the moment when one starts wondering what link there might be between nothing in particular and what is going on in the room, what the child is doing. At other times, one may vaguely follow the child's play, suggest a new direction it might take, or teasingly do something disruptive. At such a moment, the mode of thought is akin, in its indeterminacy, to the way an analyst listens. You become what I once termed the "drowsy nanny." Though a nanny knows how to doze while still being aware of what is going on, at the same time she is able to keep a mental distance between herself and the child in her charge. In those circumstances, something peculiar happens to communication: it can still take place between two living beings, except that it is inadvertent. This sort of exchange can sometimes have the effect of making the child suspend her compulsive repetitions. Then, at other moments, the therapist's thoughts become more defined, for example, if the child's procedures show a sudden variation. One wants to see what it is that has changed and why, so one starts to think in terms of linguistics or cognitive science. The mode of thought has changed; the waiting goes on.

How Do You Speak to a Child without Language?

As an adult, how can you speak to a child who does not speak to you? It all depends on which adult you are, the relation you have with your own history as a child, your mood of the moment, your therapeutic assumptions, whatever you may imagine about the child and his difficulties, and whatever notions you can glean about the child's emotional and mental responses to his encounter with you. This list is as eclectic as one of Jacques Prévert's poetic inventories and does not aim at being exhaustive. My impression is, though, that the way one speaks to a child is also affected by where you both are: I have had occasion to leave my consulting room and take a child down to a local park, and I am pretty sure that my ways of speaking to the same child in the two different places were not the same.

As for style, it has to conform first and foremost to some of the desiderata of a good dialogue between mother and child. Personally, I make an effort to keep my delivery slow, my vocabulary simple, and my sentences short (seldom more than four words) and to use more dramatic intonations and delivery (both by broadening the range of my variations from my basic speaking voice and by the length of my pauses). I also take care to let the substance be conveyed by the affect, even if it is descriptive. The same goes for the form I contrive to give to the linking of our exchanges: many of my statements start by taking up something the child has said; whenever possible, I try to comment on the child's words, to enrich them, or to make them more precise.

However, I do not have a single style. It depends entirely on the child I am addressing. If a child declines to make eye contact, I do not try to establish it; if a child speaks in an unmodulated voice, so do I; if a child mixes up the pronouns "I" and "you," I avoid using them; if a child's usage is halting or inaccurate, then I try to speak in allusions. Nor do I keep talking to a child who is playing: I see no virtue in intensive exposure of children to language. Often I utter only a few monosyllables, as long as they are unambiguous and directly linked to what is going on between us, to what we are feeling and experiencing. Above all (unlike most of these children's mothers), I am careful not to require anything of them. I wish to avoid putting them in any situation where they might take my tone of voice to mean that I expect a reply. I rule out both ordering and questioning. My words are never a way of trying to make this or that child do something (this, by the way, marks me off in no small measure from the way these children are spoken to by most of the adults in their lives). What I do try to do is to underscore what happens between us, offer a comment on it, not unlike what the chorus does in Greek tragedy: if a toy sheep falls, I may accompany its accident with a "Boom"; if all the things have now been taken out of the toybox, I may make the point by adding "Done" or "There." So my first words do not contain either questions or orders. Nor are they interpretations of what the child is doing: I do not say, "Oh, dear, you've dropped the sheep," or "Well, that sheep was really annoying you." What my words do try to do is crystallize a changed state that has come about in our shared situation. And I also try to formulate them in a way that is actually the opposite of an interpretation, a "neutral" way, without adopting any particular point of view, as though it is something that the child and I can both see in the same way, as though I am just putting into words a thought that might belong to one or other of us. So speech uttered in the presence of the child is speech not addressed to the child. It must not be addressed to the child: if it infringes that rule, it becomes an interruption, an intrusion, an incursion. If there is to be a circulation of words, one must try not to hold on to them, so that whatever is said sounds rather like some nameless song overheard through an open window, sung by the voice of someone forgotten. At this stage, language is basically little more than a way of marking an alteration in the landscape, of identifying a discontinuity and constructing it as an object. In addition, of course, it is an indirect way of laying the foundations for possible generalization from the present situation. If I make a point of saying "Boom" not only when the sheep falls but when anything else falls, I think I am helping the child to create a kind of preconception of a fall, regardless of the type of object that falls, whether it is a sheep, an elephant, or a lump of plasticine. In this way, the spoken word can help the child toward a sort of division of the real, by separating the idea of a fall from all the other infinite contingencies to which it is of necessity connected. My "Boom" progressively brings the child to see the outcome of the fall as a stable state resulting from a process. Onomatopoeias of this kind foster the child's ability to see different objects as going together and to make categories. By saying "Knock, knock" each time one knocks on doors as dissimilar as an office door and the swing door out in the corridor, one is promoting the child's ability to construct a commonality, a sort of "preconcept" or "precategory," which will serve to bring together objects that in other respects are not assimilable to one another. Then, a little later on, when I decide to hide the plasticine that the child wants to roll into balls, if I just say "Plasticine?" at the very moment when I can see from her eyes that she is looking in the box for the thing I have put somewhere else without her knowing, then this is another way of helping her to crystallize a thought content, because it also lets her see that I was able to interpret the meaning of her glance, that I understood what she wanted, and that we are in fact thinking about the same thing.

The Work Session

A work session with children without language is, strictly speaking, neither a session of psychotherapy (I mostly say nothing, though I take an active part in play), a session of speech therapy, nor a session of belated mothering. My most pressing concern is to eschew any inappropriate schoolteacherly behavior, so as to let the child (re)claim the role of a subject with something meaningful to say. By being present at the child's play, I aim constantly to supply a simplified mirror of what he does spontaneously or to offer him a possible way of elaborating it. The purpose is to create a space for exchange and communication without having any necessarily linguistic focus. In good cases, this enables the child to establish a mode of communication comparable to what one can see in normal children between nine and fourteen months; and eventually there is exchange for the sake of exchange, for the pleasure of it, for a game: do/undo, tie/untie, hold on/let go, taking turns, then taking turns again, for weeks on end.

In Praise of Repetition

In the best cases, as the sessions pass, our time together gradually falls into set sequences which are pretty well marked off from one another. The child selects a few centers of interest, each of them the focus of a series of actions, which are all organized into a fixed order. For example, he will make for the lump of plasticine, go through his ritual of pulling pieces off it to roll into balls before molding them all back together in a single mass. As our sessions progress, this sequence of actions becomes a routine centered on a particular emblematic object within that segment of the session. In addition to the plasticine, other objects (a toy car, but also the window or the door, for example) become the organizing focus of a segment.

What is the meaning that develops in the course of any given routine? First and foremost, for the child, going through the same motions with the same objects week after week is a way of being reassured and of feeling almost bodily that, despite my absence between sessions, I really am just the same as I was the last time: doing the same actions means that nothing has changed, especially me. In addition to that reassurance, ritual also helps to build shared thinking between the two of us. When the routine has become familiar, a child who goes over to the toybox to fish out the plasticine knows what is going to happen. More important, he knows that I know it, too. This means we are both thinking of the same things at the same moment. We are almost bound to be thinking like that because of the very objects we are both attending to. Each time he takes out the lump of plasticine, he knows that I know he is about to pull bits off it and roll them into balls. And once the balls are set out in a row, we are both thinking of what is to happen next: they will all be squashed together again and made into a single lump.

In this way, within each sequence (whether it is the one with the plasticine or the set of movements he goes through with the door routine), each stage takes on a particular status. By virtue of its place in the order of events, it acquires a meaning as a sign and an indicator: it becomes the sign heralding the action to follow and the indicator of the action just done. As soon as the child starts pulling bits off the original lump, it is for both of us a material sign of his intention to make them into balls. And when the balls are made, they are not just balls: each of them represents the crystallization of the previous state, when they were just random bits of plasticine picked off the big lump. In a sense, the result of each stage of any ritual stands as a retrospective sign for the stage just past and an anticipatory one for the stage coming next. In this way, routines and their ritualization serve as the adjunct for accession to semiotic functioning.

As can be appreciated, for each segment of a routine to constitute a true object of thought, more is required than that the routine just be stabilized into differentiated sequences. It is also necessary for it to achieve a degree of autonomy. This requires work, a process in which the therapist's attitude can function as a catalyst. Of primary importance is the adult's attentiveness to the child's activity. A child playing with plasticine all alone in his own room at home and a child playing with plasticine in the presence of an adult silently watching do not act in the same way. For one thing, the very fact of passing from one game to another while an adult is there doing nothing reinforces the child's sense of self-control. For another thing, even if the adult is not doing anything, merely by looking at and paying attention to the sequence of events organized by the child he is helping each of these events to become autonomous. The child can then gradually progress toward a realization of the existence of discontinuity and of the relative autonomy of each phase; this helps the child to see each of these as a kind of object whose role is no longer just to be an obligatory element with a fixed place in a set of linked procedures.

The therapist's function is to support and develop a child's way of expressing a thought, to make it a little more complex and, at times, even to go against it, with the aim of encouraging a clearer or more accurate expression of it. In the early stages, the therapist's intention may be to just let a lull of space evolve in its own way with the hope that out of it will come a definition of what is to be the theme of the exchanges. This is brought about by the undesigned functioning of repetitions, which allows both of the participants to know where the focus of their communication will lie. Routines gradually secrete commonplaces, so one can let the repetition become stabilized. The attention one pays to its component phases helps one to see each of them as an object readily put into words. This constitutes a vital facilitation in the process of building a theme. The child learns to signal when he wants the next phase to start up. In this way, what is facilitated is the preverbal expression of an anticipation or a wish. Independently of all of that, however, the putting together of a stable and differentiated repetitive sequence contributes to the emergence of signs: in any series of phases, every event becomes a premonitory sign of the one following. A sequence becomes stable when it is based on the memory of the occurrences of the same sequence in previous sessions; the child knows that knowledge of this is knowledge shared. The meaning that attaches to an event seen by two pairs of eyes as belonging to a series is that of an announcement of a coming event (or a reminder of the one before). The set nature of every stage of the series means that each of them acquires the status of a signifier corresponding to two signifieds: the stage after and the stage before. A sign has been created: a visible signifier (a hand movement) can be related to an invisible signified (the event just past or the one just to come). A possibility of communication has also been created: there now exists a frame for it; and speech can start to punctuate the recurring rhythms of its stages. Too often, though, repetitions can become too fixed. In such cases, a judicious touch of conflict or a little designed impediment to the rerunning of the set scenario, by requiring a child to express a desire with greater vigor, may prove useful in prompting the development of linguistic behaviors. Experience shows that children do not make the effort required by the self-representation of things (to bring them first to representation, then to words) unless they are confronted by a disparity between what was expected to happen and what happens—when, for instance, you expect to find a thing in its proper place but the place is empty. By slightly inflecting an accustomed practice, one can sometimes help bring about a representation requiring words.

Constructing Objects of Thought

Of the ways the adult can transform a stage of ritual into a (relatively) independent object of thought, there are some that are much more direct than mere glances. For example, one can simply prevent the action that defines the stage. Faced with the impediment, the child has to construct a representation of what she cannot achieve. In so doing, she sees it as a project, an aim, the outcome of a design. In this way, a stage that until then has been little more than an automatic mark in the series of stages becomes a real object of thought, identified as such and with autonomous status.

Clearly, no such deliberate upsetting of an established order of proceedings should be attempted until the regularity of the exchanges between adult and child has given a sure basis on which to gradually inflect things. And this may take many months. Also, the success of each attempt can be measured only by the way the child reacts, one's purpose being of course not to prevent her from doing what she wants to do but to prompt her to persevere despite the detour put upon her. Prompting like this goes hand in hand with a sort of gentle teasing. In most games, there comes a moment when, instead of giving the child what she needs, I play hard to get, as though I want her to talk me into it. The result of this can often be that a child has to clarify what she wants me to do, and the meaning gesture may become more explicit. To take the plasticine example again, rather than handing it to her when I feel she is about to ask for it, I leave it inside a closed box that is clearly visible so that she has to show her intention of using the plasticine, or even has to point at the box in a manner that is more or less purposeful. In other circumstances, my strategy will be not to feign deliberate uncooperativeness but to slightly complicate the physical parameters of her situation in a way that obliges her, if she is to achieve her desired result, to alter the sequence of her spontaneous acts. This means that I may, very visibly, "hide" the stick of plasticine under the table, thus obliging the child to fetch it from a place other than its usual one in the box. The point of all these scenarios is to build in minor variations to the basic script, not so as to prevent the child from carrying out her project but with the object of making her accommodate a deviation, a new turn of things that complicates her familiar arrangements. And, of course, if she manages to do this, it will also help to reinforce in her whatever sense of self she may have.

Thought-Controlling the Adult's Mind

By and large, everything I have described derives from the play and actions of the child as seen by both child and adult, as in the case of the plasticine. There are, however, other games in which the adult's behavior is more directly inflected by the child and for which I use the notion of thought control. The point of these games is simple: to have the child grasp the idea that he is manipulating the mind of the person he is addressing, to have him understand that the mind is a living thing (exactly like his own in that respect) but that he can activate it or deactivate it at will. What gives value to this game is this very alternation between the animate state and the inanimate. In these circumstances, the adult becomes a sort of live puppet under thought control.

When a child agrees to play with the idea that he can activate another person's body the way he can an inert object (a toy car, for instance, that he can push along), the otherness of others' thinking becomes bearable. The thing that is fundamentally important here is that the adult must be under thought control and not manual control. There is a difference: manual control occurs when an autistic child who wants to leave a room whose door is closed takes hold of the adult's hand and puts it on the doorknob so that he will turn it. The child lays a hand on the adult's body; he initiates the desired movement in the hope that the rest will follow. Generally, there is no symbolic effect in this, for the adult is a mere instrument. If he fails to open the door, the child gets angry; if he does open it, the child dashes out. In either case, the motor release that follows the request cancels any thinking. Nor does the adult offer at any moment a representation of the child's purpose, by, say, miming the movement of a door opening. However, another child may take intense pleasure not only in working a swing door but also in seeing the adult start to imitate a swing door, by swaying from side to side in time with its movements. This is the situation that I call thought control: the child activates an inert object, the door, and the adult imitates not the child but the object that the child has activated. In other words, he is showing himself to the child as an object that can be activated or deactivated at will. Through this type of game, the child realizes that he can influence the mind of another person, which in return alters considerably the notion he has of the thoughts, the affects, the representations, and the identity of that person.

What has to be done, for quite a long time, is to accept the place given to you by the child, though this may entail spending many long hours in a loop of repetitions. You become the thing of the child. I spent months writing down the names of foods dictated by a child; walking around the corridors of the Alfred Binet Center, session after session, in accordance with a strictly identical itinerary; blowing in the ear of a little boy in the hope that he would eventually turn toward me to have me do it again. The essential thing is that the child must gradually become able to fit the adult into his ritual. The next thing is that he must come to an acceptance of variations. And the final one is that he must come to see meaning in the events caused by the other person.

I have often wondered what it is in so many children without communication or language that gives them this need for control, this singular way they have of imposing their will on an adult. I suspect it represents an attempt to deprive the other person of autonomy of sound and movement, these being, in living things, the most perceptible signs of autonomy of thought. And, as we know, autonomous thought is insufferable. It is the source of the nasty things others do to us: because they can think for themselves, they can drop out of a game, go away, leave us to our aloneness. Autonomy of sound and movement, which are the signs of autonomous thought, is the dreadful mark of a constant ability to leave. That is why we have this natural hatred for the thinking of someone else, and very often for all thinking. If children are ever to partake in exchange, it is obviously crucial that they get over this initial way of feeling, so as to find pleasure in dealings with others. And that can often start with the illusion of exercising thought control over them.

Squiggles, a First Written Sign

Throughout the sessions with these children, I am constantly trying to create a communicative space for signs. Signs can crop up quite without warning. Sometimes all that is required is to draw a child's attention to the mark left by an act. If, for instance, a child sits squiggling randomly on a piece of paper, and if the adult then reproduces the same pencil movements and marks, the child may look closely at the result. If exchanges can then focus on what has been drawn, one has stepped into the realm of meaning, for a mark left by a pencil is a very first signifier: whether for the adult or for the child, it always implies the action that made it. The signifier is a squiggle, and its signified is the squiggling.

This exchange through squiggling is in some respects similar to the squiggle game that Winnicott played with his child patients. However, my perspective is rather different. Winnicott's aim was to collaborate with the child in a shared creation that was to lead to an exchange through speech. Given that the children I deal with do not speak, my own purposes are much less ambitious: to bring them to see something interesting in the result of their act of squiggling and to show them that in the mark left on the paper, in the squiggle itself, I can make out different shapes, each one of which corresponds to a different action. This type of interaction does presuppose, however, a measure of openness in the child; it is unusual for it to emerge in the earliest stages. The child must first come to an acceptance of the adult's involvement in his act.

Side by Side and Face to Face

Despite their repetitiveness, their extreme simplicity, and their at times minimal character, these ritualized games do not all serve the same purpose. To my mind, they engage with two categories of symbolic functions that are radically different from one another. In the first of them, each of the participants sits or stands opposite the other, and they take turns. There is a clear distinction between the two positions, and each of the players can occupy them at different times. So the positions are not just opposed; they are also complementary. This is the sort of turn-taking play that is commonly observed in the young child who learns, for example, to catch a ball thrown by his mother, to throw it back to her, then to catch it again when it is thrown back to him. The second of the categories consists of games in which both the adult and the child are looking in the same direction. In these cases, they are "side by side." This type of play helps to enrich and stabilize joint attention. The child and the adult become used to building a shared theme for future exchange. There is an atmosphere of undefined consensus. What is most important is that they share the feeling of a certain single-mindedness, which exchange will be able to elaborate and give a sharper focus to.

An Example of Play Side by Side

After dark, we see the headlights of cars passing on the roadway outside. As the child is looking at them, I start to speak of the way they come along the street, pass in front of us, then slide away from us and eventually disappear. If by saying something like "Gone" each time a car disappears around the corner I can calm the child's anxiety, then a side-by-side exchange is under way. When we both have our noses to the window-pane, neither of us is looking at the other. All I am doing is focusing my own eyes on what she is interested in: both pairs of eyes are gazing at the same object, a car. Importantly, it is an object that neither of us is handling, that is out of reach of both of us. For once, this puts us on an equal footing. This situation is, of course, rather frustrating, but that is the very reason that the comments I voice on the appearance then the disappearance of the vehicle become a kind of magic attempt to alleviate our shared impotence at the thing of light that comes then goes. The spoken words give a rhythm to the glimpse we get of some inaccessible and faraway place, a place that neither of us can have any purchase on, except through thinking about it. In such moments of play-sharing, the child's interest, slowly and not without a perceptible reluctance, tilts away from the inaccessible object toward the ritualized word game growing out of the three stages of the headlights' appearing, their passing in front of us, and then their gradual disappearance at the end of the street. The cars can appear and disappear at will, but language is our only recourse against our lack of power to act on them: it gives meaning to what is happening; it actually makes one imagine what is about to happen, especially if the ritual is consolidated by the repetitions. When it is dark and two watchers are standing at a window, if what both are seeing is put into speech by one of them, that changes what is perceived into a signifying indicator. In that sense, just looking jointly at a shape is incipient symbolization.

When the adult and the child are looking in the same direction and one of them speaks of what they are both watching, speech arises in an indefinite continuum between them. We both know which of us is speaking, but what is said expresses our combined attention. Since either of us can add a comment on the thing seen, the continuum of thought enables alternation of roles and the eventual emergence of a distinction between who is speaking and who isn't. As will be readily understood, "side by side" refers not to a merely spatial relationship but to a symbolic position that may be adopted in dialogue and that can be defined as follows: the adult does not try to address the child; the adult does not wish to make the child a target for spoken words. So I just let my words lie, as it were, somewhere between us, in case the child should bother or feel inclined—or not, as the case may be—to take them up. In that way, I feel, speech can have an effect, by letting the child experience the words as though they might have come from either of us, as though I were somehow merely the casual and accidental voicer of an exchange and a thought that go on belonging to both of us. This is why, wherever we happen to be in my room, I often speak to the child as though making asides. To make these asides sound as though spoken by either of us, I try to avoid direct speech, face to face, so as not to confront him with my words. It is this mode of sidelong speech, as it were, that I mean when I define our respective exchange positions as "side by side." Psychoanalysts trained in the use of psychodrama may see this way of speaking as reminiscent of the way a psychodramatist sometimes adopts the role of a patient's "double" and gives voice to what he or she is thinking. However, in my view, this is a faulty analogy. "Doubling," putting someone else's thoughts into words, is speaking on the person's behalf, using the words we imagine the person might use. What we say, though, is spoken not for ourselves but for the other person. Side-by-side speech, in contrast, consists of putting into words thoughts that, though suspended, are somewhere in the exchange between us, thoughts that hardly belong more to one of us than to the other. It expresses thoughts that are interstitial, intermediary, and transitional, ungrounded, without a definite source.

The Presence of Winnicott

On the whole, the children I deal with suffer from a mode of psychic discontinuity caused by an unremitting agitation that prevents them from ever playing properly. Their needs, their urges, their desires are so strong and so disparate that they live amid an emotional torrent that deprives them of the stability required to exercise thought on what happens to them and to sense in themselves any ongoing center for their own affects. The real difficulty is that the adult who is with them is as much a cause of agitation as a source of reassurance. If things are to change for the better, the child must come to find the required stability in the adult's constant interest in him. But the knowledge that he has no control over what happens to him aggravates his anxiety. If things are to change, the therapist must stop being a person and turn into an atmosphere. According to Winnicott, who speaks of this in relation to the mother of the very young infant, she has to fulfil two functions. Firstly, by giving herself to the child as an object of love and hatred, she accepts his urges. In this way, she is a source not only of life and movement but of conflict and torment.

Secondly, though, she must also be an atmosphere, a caring environment capable of protecting the child from too strong agitation and facilitating the construction of a basis through which to mentally process the love and hatred that he directs at his mother as an object (Winnicott 1957). The problem for the therapist is that the mother as atmosphere is the same person who provides everyday physical care, the one who tends to bodily needs and all aspects of mothering; the functions of the therapist do not correspond to any of that. Now and again I may take a child to the bathroom or help to change one who has wet himself, but this happens so seldom that it could never serve as the basis for the construction of the child's narcissism. There is, however, this other means of side-by-side play. In an attempt to reduce the agitation a child may feel in my presence, I avoid facing him. When we are face to face, awareness of what distinguishes us from each other is sharper and more pressing. But when we sit side by side, the marking of what makes us separate and different is a nonproblem. With the interest I take in what the child is seeing, I am not so much a mirror for his identity as a simple adjunct to the fact that he is looking at something.

Toward Indistinctness in Exchange

According to some theories, communication (and speech too, for that matter) can happen only if one feels distinct from the person one is speaking to. Any refusal to feel individuated makes it impossible. The process of individuation is a painful one; sometimes a child's refusal to engage in exchange may be a way of avoiding it. Here, too, the side-by-side arrangement allows for another way of engaging in exchange, without imposing the precondition that there be separateness and an absolute differentiation between interlocutors.

I am not trying to present side-by-side play as a cure-all. In many cases, you can stare for hours at whatever it is that holds the child's interest without the slightest thing happening. I am trying not to describe a method of reeducation but just to draw attention to certain unsuspected advantages that can derive from engaging with some of the child's most straightforward and spontaneous movements, on condition that it be done unobtrusively. Engagement with a child's perception in this way gives it the quality of an exchange, even though such exchange entails a definite measure of illusion and misunderstanding. What one may have shared with the child may not become apparent until much later, on the day, for example, when he starts talking while looking out of the window or saying something about things that appear then disappear, or things that come and go then come back. When that happens, one is bound to wonder and to see with hindsight that something did come of the perception that was shared.

5

From Communication to Language

Up to now, I have spoken of the creation of a space for communication as above all an attempt to build joint attention. This element is essential. The ability to cope with sharing of attention, to accept thinking jointly without feeling overwhelmed by the presence of the other person, is a necessary condition for the later growth of exchange.

When it comes to language, this prerequisite of communication leaves its mark on the content of what is spoken. From a linguistics perspective, most utterances can be analyzed into a base form in two parts: the topic and the comment (sometimes referred to as theme and rheme). A topic consists of a set of words functioning as a definer of the zone of shared ground that the rest of the utterance aims to specify. The topic gives the listener a hint about what is going to be said, roughing out the broad area of relevance while narrowing it down and setting it within a framework. By definition, the topic has to remain approximate enough not to exhaust the statement at one go. There is a clear difference between the use of words in a topic and their use in a comment: topic words are used as pointers to a shared field of thought, with a function analagous to that of objects one simultaneously points at and looks at, whereas comment words make precise and explicit what it is that the speaker wishes to express within that field. A simple example would be to say, "Speaking of fish, I love sole," a statement in which the topic ("Speaking of fish") sets out a field of thought that is clear as to subject matter, though still rather unclear as to detailed reference: the speaker might be going on to talk of fishing instead of cooking; and what is coming remains unknown. So the topic establishes common ground for the exchange that is to follow. It is on this basis that the comment ("I love sole") then clarifies the content that the speaker wishes to bring to the attention of the listener. In the comment, a speaker expresses his or her personal addition to the topic. With the comment ("I love sole"), thought is given expression through determinate words.

Broadly speaking, in order to achieve full expression as a comment, thought must progress through three different stages. First, it must contrive to single out stable segments from the continuous stream of sensations and perceptions. Next, these segments must be given a profile corresponding to one of the three basic linguistic formats: verb (process), patient, and agent. And then it must reassemble this trio of profiles within a propositional content. A comment is made of this content.

Putting Together Topic and Comment

By the time any child can contrive to make a statement of two words, the topic/comment linkage is definitively established. For example, if a child sees a cat leaving via a window and says merely "Gone!," it may be nothing more than an automatic speech movement, expressing surprise and disappointment. If, however, the statement is "Gone cat!," then there is a change not only in speech form but also in thought. To make such a statement, the child must be able to think in two ways about the cat's leaving and then combine them. She starts by reducing the whole situation to an event—leaving—and this is what makes her say "Gone!" The second stage consists of reviewing the situation as expressed in the initial unspecified form and conveying another version of it focused not on the situation as event but on the essential organizing agent of it. In her complete utterance, there are in fact two successive profilings of a single content of thought, two successive ways of making it into a sort of metonymy: first, by a definition of the event that happens (i.e., a disappearance, noted as "Gone"), and then by a definition of the topic involving the disappearance ("cat"). These can be said to constitute two versions of a single change that has happened in the world. The first version focuses on the disappearance, the occurrence that has come to pass; the second focuses on the central topic, the cat. Each of the two words derives from a separate way of envisaging the whole and gives an abstract of it, a metonymy. But each of them is also a way of specifying what the other one has left unspecified. A prerequisite for any disappearance is something that disappears, and on that,

"Gone" has nothing to say, unlike "cat," which defines the object of the disappearance. The ability to speak two words thus presupposes the ability to think simultaneously about a single situation from more than one point of view, or, to put it another way, the ability to see things from a perspective other than one's own. One must also retain in the mind both versions of what one wants to speak of, without one of them canceling out the other. One must be able to think of the occurrence both as a sudden departure and as something bearing essentially on a cat. In addition, the speaker must be capable of going beyond simple reformulation, given that "cat" is not mere supplementary information on the nature of the disappearance. In fact, the representation of the situation seen as concerning the agent (the situation as related to the cat) and the representation of the situation seen as concerning the event (the departure) have to be put together in a way that is different from that required by mere supplementary information. The speaker must specify the link between the two ways of seeing what is being spoken of and not just place them in apposition to each other. To put it another way, the relation between agent and activity (or instrument and activity, or activity and result) must be structured and then marked in the sound chain by an appropriate grammatical marker.

As can be seen, a situation in the world cannot be reduced to verb, subject, and object. To begin with, it is a whole, and the verb, the subject, and the object represent three differing "versions" of it. One has to grasp the relations among them, then express these through organized syntax. When these different operations have been mastered, the language used is no longer automatic but has become "intentional." And speech that is intentional means that a speaker, without actually noticing it, can not only cope with thinking from various angles but can fit these angles together.

Normally, this ability to think from diverse perspectives comes in successive stages. A first stage occurs when a signifier may have been given different meanings, for example, when a child says "Bye-bye" both at a moment when she is leaving (or when something disappears) and at a moment when she wants to leave (or wants something to disappear). If she says it with two different intonations, this of itself implies that she is capable of seeing the same representation content as having two different functions. This is a first level of thinking from different perspectives. The second level, that of juxtaposition, is attained when the child can repeat a statement in which she varies the order of the words, making it either "Why baby eating?" or "Baby eating, why?" or even "Baby, why eating?" However, the full level of intentional speech is not reached until a single object of thought can be seen from different angles and the relation between these angles can be specified.

Constructing a Comment

Up to now, I have been stressing the way in which therapeutic work develops and builds up joint attention and how pointing at things can make them into indicators akin to the words that state the topic in an utterance. I want now to speak of the games through which a child can become familiar with the three prototypes that enable the ideas in a comment to be expressed.

Everyday life subjects human beings to an uninterrupted flow of sensations, perceptions, affects, urges, and variations. It is difficult to say where one of these ends and another begins. The ancient Greeks defined speech as splitting things into parts, as division into segments. This entails, of course, a division of the signifier into syllables, but also a division of experience. In order to speak, human beings have to be able to split their experience of life into segments and to give an outline to the things that are to be spoken. They must also be able to fit these things into forms that correspond to the different categories known as verbs, animate nouns, and inanimate nouns. There are children who apparently either lack this ability to fragment and to format or who do not spontaneously draw on it in communication. The setting in place of categories such as verb (process), agent, and patient can be aided by certain types of play, which are additional to those suited to developing joint attention (and establishment of topics). Play of this sort can often consist of very simple manipulations. Unlike some educative procedures devised for infants in their first months of life, these activities do not develop any particular cognitive ability. They do not aim, for example, at fostering awareness of shapes, sounds, or colors. Also, they are mostly initiated by the children and require lengthy repetition, sometimes over a period of weeks or months. I usually keep out of things, trying mainly to ritualize phases of activity and to structure contrasts. For me, the really important thing is to watch. I am convinced that the child's motor and perceptive efforts are given a focus by this watching. In my presence, the child's action is not done solely for her own sake. Nor is it done wholly for my sake, but it is done as I watch. In this way, differences are established, then stabilized, and she may bring these up later in exchange. The cognitive domain becomes engaged through the meaningfulness of the exchange; motor function and perception become organized through the sharing of a representation and an affect.

Concretely, all abstract games function through a single mode of alternation, that between two states. The paradigm is "Peekaboo": first the teddy is visible, then it disappears behind the mother's back. This is the same alternation between two states as we see in playing at running a toy car across the floor to an adult, who sends it back, or when the child enjoys pulling a small piece off a lump of plasticine, then squashing it all together again. In such play, the attention is constantly focused on the alternating contrasts: now you see the teddy, now you don't; the car is pushed away, then it comes back; the piece of plasticine is separate, then joined to the lump. The game consists of deforming the way you see an object, by removing, then replacing one of its essential features. In each case, this feature corresponds to a property that is characteristic of the linguistic category being used by the child. With the teddy, for instance, the pair consists of "being there/not being there." It is a pair that involves the idea of time, which is integral to the category of the verb. With the plasticine play, what is central is the whole/part relation: it is seen in the grammar of nouns, in the difference between nouns that are countable (such as "ball": to quantify it, one speaks of "a ball" and not "some ball") and those that are uncountable (such as "plasticine": in quantifying, one speaks of "some plasticine" and not "a plasticine"). Basically, the games we play remain abstract, with very little representation of anything. They require neither characters nor any simulation of human activity, such as drinking or washing. They are the antithesis of the kind of children's play one is used to, where a child will make two puppets have a fight or kiss one another, lay out a tea set to pretend to have a meal, sit a little articulated figure on a chair or make a crocodile bite it. Such anthropomorphized play expresses a story that can be scripted. It makes reference to scenes from real life or fantasy life, images, situations, affects, and urges. The affect associated with the imaginary situations is largely responsible for the pleasure afforded by this play, much more so than the actions it involves. In abstract games, conversely, the source of pleasure is the very motor activity of the child, as well as the alternation between two different states, which is the reason for this activity. This alternation is always close to a paradigm of tension/relaxation. The whole point seems to consist in the two movements and their endless repetition: with one movement, something is there, and with the other, nothing is there; with one movement, something is done, and with the other, something is undone. What is important is the manipulation of an aspect of things almost independent of the object through which it becomes manifest: there/not there, apart/together, in/out, open/closed, lit/unlit. Whatever the activity, either one of the two states is no more than the negation of its opposite. So alternation brings out the feature around which thought has to shape itself if it is to become utterable. The content of such manipulations is infinitely variable, but there are always three main prototypes: verb, patient, agent. What has to be done is to bring out the features that characterize each of these categories. This can sometimes lead to surprises, for example, the fact that, for a child, what defines an agent is autonomy of sound and movement: what agent "means" is having the ability to move and make sounds unaided.

The Verb

My thoughts on the value of these games come essentially from observation, as well as from occasional discussions among colleagues who work either in psychoanalysis or linguistics. They also owe something to Jerome Bruner's work on spontaneous play between mother and child (see especially Bruner 1983). And they coincide with some propositions from Antoine Culioli's enunciative linguistics (Culioli 1990), as well as with the views of certain scholars in cognitive linguistics (Lakoff & Johnson 1980, Langacker 1987). As is well known, one of the theories underlying cognitive linguistics is the relation posited between certain major syntactical categories of language (notably time, space, and the subject-verb-object link) and invariables in the registers of perception and motor activity. From this point of view, the various abstract games I am about to describe seem to me to confirm the idea that notional forms such as verb, patient, and agent do correspond to prototypes that grow out of play activity that children develop spontaneously, as though they have to prepare their minds for acceding to linguistic forms. Some games do help children to acquire a kind of intuitive (or practical) knowledge of what a verb, a patient, and an agent are. As will be seen, in each of these games, the children focus their manipulation on one of the characteristic dimensions of the category, first trying to impart it to an object, then to remove it.

Games of the "peekaboo" variety, for example, contribute to laying the foundations of the idea of verb (or process). Others exercise various aspects of the category of noun.

Two Perspectives on Time

The idea that underlies verbs is time. Despite what is commonly thought to be the case, time as it functions in language is not reducible just to the distinctions among present, past, and future. What it offers is a point of view on the world, organized in two rather different ways. The first of these we use to give meaning to what we see of the world as we speak of it, in relation to a project that, depending on the grammatical form used, may be completed or only begun (uncompleted). For example, if there are a few crumbs on the table beside a used cup and I say, "I've had breakfast," the meaning I give to this situation is that it is the result of a project, namely to have breakfast. If, on the other hand, I say, "I'm having breakfast," this is a way of saying that what you see me doing can be clarified if you see it as a project undertaken but not yet completed. In each case, the grammatical form used (perfect tense or present) gives meaning to what is visible in the present situation by saying something about the state of the project of having breakfast. The second of time's two functions in language is rather different, in that it is used to allude to invisible events and to relate them to one another. It fixes the time frame of a narrative or the stages of a purpose. This can be seen in statements like "Yesterday, I had breakfast at seven o'clock and then went out for a ride on my bike," or "Next Sunday, I'm going to have breakfast at seven o'clock and then go out for a ride on my bike." In both statements, the system is identical: the breakfast and the ride are two events seen as points in time, which are related by the order of the words. Here, the intention is not to make sense of a present situation but rather to make a relation between facts that are themselves unrelated to the state of the world as we speak of them.

Time Games

Each of these two different time perspectives fits with games of different sorts. The completed/uncompleted perspective clearly belongs with "peekaboo" games: when you invest what you see with the meaning of a project completed or uncompleted, then you are thinking in terms identical to those which structure games of appearing and disappearing, and which will express themselves in words such as "there," "gone," or "again." These words speak of the world as a place where projects are accomplished, either already undertaken or soon to be undertaken.

In the case of the mother who keeps showing the teddy, then hiding it behind her back for a time, when it meets the child's eye it becomes the result of a project of appearing. This result is stable, since it can remain present until the mother and the child decide to make it disappear again.

There are other, more rudimentary games that the adult can turn into time play, although on the face of it they do not involve time. For instance, if a child stands there swaying his body nonstop from side to side, then, unlike in the teddy game, there is never a moment at which a stable state occurs; when the child stops swaying, no result has been achieved. Nevertheless, the child's movement involves recurrence; the adult can stress this recurrence with a verbal accompaniment, saying "Tick" when the child sways to the right and "Tock" when he sways to the left. This is one way among a great many to underline the existence of two transitory and opposite states, "swaying to the right" and "swaying to the left." The contrast between them, unstable though it is as a movement, becomes stable through the link with speech. One may even have to invent phases where there are none, after the manner of a colleague of mine who, in dealing with an autistic child who kept on spinning around, had the idea of clapping her hands each time he was facing her. This way of introducing discontinuity into his incessant circular movement led to some interesting progress.

So there are games that work by virtue of the contrast between two stable states, and there are others in which the adult must take a hand to mark the existence of the phases. This marking can frequently develop into a turn-taking game of its own.

In addition to all these games that familiarize children with the time dimensions of the completed and the uncompleted, there are others that give them experience of time as chronology. These are ritualized scenario games. There are any number of possible scenarios, but they all require the existence of at least three different elements, each of which has a set place in the whole. For example, there is the one in which the child pushes a car toward the adult with the aim of knocking over a little toy figure, waits to see the figure fall and the adult stand it up again, then sees the adult run the car back to him. This makes a series of events with a meaning that can exist only through the chronology linking them, each event marking a stage that can mean something only in respect to the stages that precede and follow. The idea of time that this uses is the one to be seen in the making of a narrative: it requires consecutiveness of separate actions, each of which is temporary and draws its importance solely from the fact that it happens before this one and after that one.

Animate, Inanimate

In abstract games of the second group, essential in my view, children's play is about ideas such as animate agent and inanimate patient.

In the case of agents, as we know, children very early on take a particular interest in animals but also in mechanical objects endowed with autonomy of sound and movement (Dennett 1991).[1] They are intrigued by this living quality: to be alive, as seen from the outside, is to have the autonomous ability to make sounds or move of one's own accord toward a chosen goal. Also, very quickly children's fascination with this leads them to make up games focused on the particular dimension of autonomous mobility: they push toy cars across the floor or roll balls so that they cover ground, then come to a stop. This makes a game on the animate/inanimate pair, as the car or the ball moves by itself, as though with autonomy of movement, as though it is an object that has been given a life of its own. Then it becomes stationary again, loses that property, and the whole process has to be repeated.

Countable, Uncountable

As well as the games that involve objects made "active" and animate, there are others that involve objects that remain inanimate. This inanimate category usually concerns distinctions between countables and uncountables. This is the difference, for example, between sand and marbles: you can count marbles, but not sand. From a cognitive point of view, this distinction is in part grounded in the fact that a marble,

1. With such objects, however, the child's game concerns giving them their autonomy of movement, then letting it run down; thus, it consists of making them animate, then letting them become inanimate.

unlike sand, has a stable contour. And the theme that structures many children's games is the testing of the contours and the identity of an object. During the game, the child's actions are focused on the individuation of the object: it is changed from being discernible to being undiscernible, from being individuated to being unindividuated. A bit of plasticine is pulled off the lump, rolled into a little ball, and placed inside a box, as a marble might be. Having started as a piece without shape or individuality, it is gradually given a contour that individualizes it and makes it countable. Each stage it passes through endows it with qualities that make it into an entity more and more independent of the original lump. But, at the end of the process, the little balls consecutively shaped are taken out, squashed together, and molded back into a single mass in which all individuation is abolished.

There are substances, such as water, that clearly do not lend themselves to individuation. Water, with its lack of either contour or resistance, is the paradigm of the uncountable object, devoid of outer shell or inner individuality, that can be forever deformed and divided up at will. Hence the passionate interest it inspires in autistic children.

The play dimension of these formatting activities lies in the variations and deformations wrought in the status given to the thing being utilized. The child plays at adding, then subtracting, the feature that means that the thing played with belongs to the format in question. If the game is being played with an individuable object, then the child will give it, then take away from it, the qualities that are the mark of its individuation. If the game is being played with an object that can be animated, then the child will provide it with the energy required to give the illusion of autonomy of movement, before letting the illusion cease and reveal an inert object.

A Generalization

In order for an event as minor as the appearing and disappearing of a car on a street, fiddling with a piece of plasticine, or something of that sort, to be the starting point for a movement toward organization, it must fit within a particular frame that is both stable and a little out of the ordinary, a ritualized space that marks a difference from the child's other everyday doings and gives a separate status to what is done there. For the children I deal with, such a status is of course afforded by the regularity of our sessions in my consulting room and the fact that I am always there. It is the unchanging setting, along with the repetition, that give the events their salience. However, in order to serve as indicators of process, patient, and agent, the play that happens there must also be varied and the contrast that marks the different phases of the child's actions must be transposable from one physical accessory to another. That is to say, decontextualization must be possible; the child must be able to replicate through other appearances and disappearances the pleasure given by the appearing and disappearing car. To this end, it is important that the games be comparable as regards their essential quality but different from one another. This can lead to a whole sequence of related activities, as in the following example taken from the appearing and disappearing games. The initial stage consisted of lengthy sessions of observation of the cars on the street below. Next there were games with a toy car, which we ran through a little tunnel made of a sheet of paper, so as to observe together the way it disappeared under the paper, then reappeared at the other end. Then, we had appearing-and-disappearing games of the more standard variety, such as opening and closing the door and hiding behind it and saying "Peekaboo" or "Bye-bye," as well as many sessions in which the child spent the whole time switching the light on and off. In this varied sequence, though the constant was obviously the contrast between presence and absence, each new situation differed from the previous one. As a sequence progressed, the child and I took a more and more active part in the effect produced. When we looked out the window, we were less active than when we ran the toy car through the tunnel. At the same time, once one of us had pushed the car, there was still something of the original watching game, as we were once again passive spectators of a disappearance and a reappearance that now depended on neither of us. Another thing: when we looked out of the window, the child and I were side by side; but when we were at opposite ends of the paper tunnel, we were facing each other. (Mind you, there are always some children who will not push the car when they are opposite me: they have to come to my end, even when we are taking it in turns to push it, as though they were incapable of doing it any other way.) So the constant being practiced was always the difference between presence and absence, though the share of both participants in each of the activities necessarily varied, as did the position they occupied in relation to each other.

In the development that I have just sketched, the type of play that is marked by rhythms such as "Peekaboo" and "Bye-bye" and the play that consists of switching the light on and off are clearly different from pushing the car. For one thing, they require total engagement of each person: the appearing and disappearing are not focused simply on a single object that is worked alternately by each of the two participants in the exchange. And for another, there is a sort of simultaneity in the disappearing and reappearing of the two of us: my encouragements, my saying "Peekaboo" and "Bye-bye," "Oh!" and "Ah!," suggest to the child that when I disappear from his sight, he too disappears from mine, even though on another level the sensation of his own body gives him a feeling of (relative) continuity.

The Effect of Games on Language

In addition to joint-attention play, games marked by rhythms and games of formatting are often the first to become established with children who have reached the age of three without speaking. They come about long before scenario games like playing with dolls or tea sets. Familiarity with abstract games seems to have a decisive effect on the starting up of language. It is as though the speech of these children is hampered by their inability to couch their thought in linguistic forms and as though such games help them to build and mobilize the missing ability. Once this type of play has been mastered, there follows a phase of intensive pointing, then the emergence of words like "phew," "good," "finished," "bye bye," "again," and "gone," each of which signals the end or the expected return of something. After that, one can see the beginnings of syntax of the sort required for expressing affect and change. One thing that remains strange is that very often there are children who do not possess this essential linguistic register, yet who do have comparatively many lexical terms and are perfectly capable of producing them, despite some difficulties of pronunciation.

Toward Figurative Play

In working with a child who does not speak, therefore, the material drawn on in the early exchanges is, by and large, rather abstract and visual in nature. To begin with, since the whole session usually passes in complete silence, it may seem rash to expect the onset of any symbolic process. And yet, after a few months, the child's play does evolve. Once we have gotten past the stage of nonfigurative manipulations, then the stages of rhythmic actions, emptying things out and putting them back in, arranging according to size and color, after the time of squiggling and ignoring the squiggles, there comes a second phase. The animals start to bite one another or to kiss, little toy people go out for a walk, and we have entered the domain of the figurative. There will of course be recurrences of abstract forms, but one can always make sense of this in terms of drive and defense mechanisms. On the whole, with this figurative mutation, there appears a new language, one that is better suited to expressing refusal, projects, and agreement, one that includes utterances such as "Baby, bathroom." And, once that happens, one can begin to make sense of the genesis of the disorder and see a clear link between representation and drive.

Very often during the course of a treatment, children eventually give up their geometrical games in favor of more standard figurative play the moment they are faced with a conflict or elaboration supplied by the therapist. This transition frequently occurs in ways that are comparable from one child to another. For example, one begins to see miming of concrete situations, such as a child pretending to have a meal with a tea set or to drink from a beaker. Here, though it is still very much a pretend action, it derives from a real situation. Then we start to witness simple imaginary figurations: a child will make a crocodile bite a toy figure. In other cases, the transition happens through a child's spontaneous reworking of the abstract play.

When these concrete games appear, they are linked to an affect or a memory; there is always a history behind them, just as there is always a scenario and a connection with human events, though these may be reduced to their simplest expression. The child's activity is the sign of a psychic conflict. The earlier alternations between two contrasting phases may have disappeared. The child's scenario becomes the metaphorical expression of a scene that is never completely realized through the game: the acting out does not exhaust the richness of what the child wants to imaginatively transpose. The imagination of the watching adult is also stimulated, which marks the beginning of a phase of speculation, the phase of make-believe. When the light is switched on, then off again, this may indicate a fantasy (e.g., sleep, darkness, nighttime, death, as opposed to daylight, activity, presence), but it now functions singly, without the breaking down into the on/off contrast. Also, the child's enjoyment now comes entirely from the ability to control light and dark. There is a different pleasure in the act of taking a toy figure, putting it into a tiny bed, then making its parents kiss it goodnight and leave it. Here, the enjoyment no longer lies in the actions themselves but in playing with the representation conjured up by the fiction enacted. So now the pleasure is not just of the unmediated sort: it is a "make-believe" pleasure.

Fostering the Figurative

It is, needless to say, difficult to isolate what produces this qualitative change from abstract play to concrete play, especially since the capacity for figurative play is very likely well established before it emerges. What one can describe, however, is the sort of tiny fluke that can set off the process. It has to do with the therapist and with a particular way he or she has of dealing with the child, as I hope to show with the following example. When a child is engaged in endlessly turning out little balls of plasticine, setting them out in a row, then putting them into a box on which he carefully puts a lid, one may be excused for feeling tempted to divert his repetitions in another direction. However, to achieve this, it would be pointless to offer him toy animals or human figures, or even to set them out on both sides of a fence and start to tell a little story about them in the hope of interesting him in the lives of animals. Nor would there be any point in taking one of his little balls of plasticine and turning it into a little person. This can certainly help to create a favorable atmosphere with many children whose difficulties are of a different kind, but it will not work with a child who does not speak and who spends his whole time doing nothing but making endless balls of plasticine. Such a child, however, is not necessarily incapable of the slightest exchange, and that is the very thing I look for. If I set out in front of him three fences in a triangle, without figures, making an enclosed space, then something may well happen. These sketchy generalities derive from a particular child I remember: he suddenly felt the urge to swap the enclosed space of the box for the enclosed space of my triangle of fences and started to transfer all his balls of plasticine. The point is that, by putting them inside the triangle, he had accepted a variation. My first idea, the one involving the human figures, would not work, but the second one, by remaining geometrical, did work. Exchange was possible between us, as long as it was geometrical in content and abstract in nature. The therapist's problem (and the fulfilment to be found in its resolution) lies in gauging how much of such variation a child will accept. One must be able to think up a possibility that is similar enough not to rule out continuing contact between us but that allows us to create something new. In the case just recounted, what swayed the child towards acceptance (at least, this is how I see it) was the fact that he liked either to set out his plasticine balls in a row (that is, in an open space) or to shut them inside a box (that is, in a closed space that makes them invisible), and the suggestion I came up with, the triangular fence, gave him a space combining two advantages: it was closed, but this did not preclude visibility. It probably gave him something of the feeling of being understood, without encroaching too much on him.

So, if it is to work, the device offered must have no overtly human or narrative features. It must be of a discreetly abstract nature; from the point of view of the child's purposes, it must also represent a "technical solution" unavailable from the results of his spontaneous activity. However, it is equally clear that, just because the child takes an interest in it, this is not a sufficient condition for having recourse to it. For, as we know, any intervention runs the constant risk of becoming in its turn the basis of a new repetitive ritual. To avoid this danger and to obviate stabilization, the device should not only be abstract but must also be capable of adaptation to the later development of a human story. This was exactly the case with the fences and the balls of plasticine. The fences can be turned into closed polygons; and they can be seen mentally as walls surrounding all sorts of things. Though the fences, like the balls of plasticine, are nonhuman objects, they are also free enough of associations to lend themselves to indeterminately human things. This is not the case, for instance, with a comb or a length of rail: they are both too constricted by and inseparable from their functional context. A length of rail is made for trains and can be used for no other purpose than to push them along in a fixed direction; a comb can be used solely for combing hair (though, if by chance a child can use it as a toy car, there is hope).

What makes fences and balls useful is that, though they are nonhuman objects, they are not too closely attached to particular contexts. They give material form to certain essential dimensions of all sorts of actions. A ball of plasticine is the outcome of a separation: you have to pull off a certain amount from the lump, and you have to reshape it. This process involves both affect and hand movement. Similarly, a set of fences arranged into a closed figure makes a mode of separation. It is, however, a separation unrelated to any particular object, whether at home, at school, or in my consulting room. What comes from using objects of this kind does not immediately amount to a human content adaptable to a narrative in stages, but that is what they can eventually lend themselves to. For instance, in the case under discussion, a little later in the session, the balls of plasticine became "toilet," and the child who spoke this word about them was thereby at the beginning of a radically new process. The conflation of feces, food, and babies (as well as the moment before, during, or after the session when the child is taken to the bathroom) can happen with these objects, and from then on they are no longer mere balls of plasticine. The scenario made its appearance when, after having played with these pieces of plasticine for a long time as though they were just that and nothing else, the child informed me that they were feces and wanted to have them disappear down the "toilet," which he asked me to construct. Here once again was the contrast between two states (balls visible as such and balls down the toilet as a single large lump), though the alternation between the separateness of the small piece of plasticine from the lump and their being stuck together again had clearly become quite marked, both as an element of a scenario and as the development of an urge. Abstract play had taken on sense in a dimension linked to bodily production. The important point here is the recycling of the abstract arrangement into a register that is more familiar to me as a childhood psychotherapist, the register of urges.

It may well be asked whether my technical device of the fences is not equivalent to a verbal interpretation in more standard treatments of children. And there is a sense, even though one of them is voiced and the other is unvoiced, in which the effects are comparable: my contribution, like a successful verbal interpretation, did enable the child to change registers, to leave his abstractions behind and step into the world of the human. But against that, abetting the action of a child and verbally interpreting actually operate in ways which are well nigh opposites. The fact is that the first effect of an accurate interpretation is to bring about a pause, a slight depression, followed by a giving up, as a prelude to the discovery of new and unsuspected horizons, whereas an initiative that merely takes up the action of a child does not lead to such a detour through depression. The unsuspected horizon is not a consequence of any giving up. With the children I treat, it is out of the question to make them give up, even momentarily. The shock of it would be too much. What is required is that any contribution crop up inadvertently, tangentially, as though it had come from nobody in particular. That it must not disturb anything is the sine qua non of its being usable by the child.

Reversal

Here is another example of a slightly different kind. In the consulting room where I see Philippe, there is a stoneware bottle. One day, when he had grabbed it and was handling it in a reckless way that bothered me, I said, "Watch this." I took it from him, put my lips to the mouth of it, and blew: the sound I made, rather like the foghorn of a ship, amused him. He took back the bottle, blew into it, and the bottle made its sound. At the next session, the bottle was completely ignored, as it was at the following one. A week later, though, it was once more the center of attention: Philippe took all the pencils and slid them one after another inside it. Then he blew into it, before going to sit on a chair, where he turned his face to the wall, lowered his head, and hid the bottle behind the chair. Eventually, he turned toward me again and told me he was sick, pointing at various orifices: a nostril, his ear, his mouth, and then his "poo-poo" (his poo-poo hurts, doing poo-poo, his anus hurts). Pain marks his recognition that his body partakes of interiority. What I see as important is that this movement appeared to derive from the episode with the bottle. It represents a singular and localized perception, as well as a turnaround of meaning for this game, which seems to have brought about the onset of the child's inner experiencing of the body as a container. By blowing into the empty bottle, I made an object of interest out of something that usually is not of interest. In general, it is full bottles that are interesting, not empty ones. Yet, in this case, what was important was that the bottle was empty, because it was only then that it could make a sound and be filled with pencils. It became the focus of a conflict: it would be nice to have it full, so as to be able to empty it; it would be nice to have it empty, so as to be able to make the sound. The conflict focused on this object of perception, though in part trivial, was enough to set off psychic change.

In chapters 4 and 5, I have referred to a range of treatments that I use with children whose pathology lies somewhere in the region of audimutism, childhood psychosis, and a particular form of less severe autism sometimes called "secondary autism." Perhaps, though, the best way to understand the links between the speech apparatus on the one hand, the broad functioning of cognitive processes on the other, and also the movements of a subject's thought and affect is to follow, step by step, certain individual treatments. Which is why I now propose to describe several of these. As luck would have it, many of the children with whom I have dealt eventually started to communicate and then to speak, although their spoken styles retained some peculiarities. I mention luck not from false modesty but from my conviction that the ideas I put forward and my therapeutic choices are anything but a cure-all. This is why, in order to shirk none of the difficulties of this endeavor and, above all, to show how complex and rich they may be, I intend to close this account of the work of therapy with an experience that, more than once, has brought me to the limits of my capacities.

Part III

Some Cases

6

Ahlem, or Painful Transparency

There are children who can reach the age of three without ever speaking. Sometimes this can be the effect of a massive personality disorder, which so badly affects nonverbal communication that all speech is made impossible. With other children, this may not be the case, even with those who seem to be taking refuge in prostration, uncontrolled agitation, or weird rituals. When I met Ahlem for the first time, she appeared to be particularly listless, though her psychological difficulties were no more severe than neurosis. Her withdrawal was so profound because it was the result of a confluence of cognitive and aphasiological problems. In fact, she was not completely averse to all contact; once she had gained a little confidence in her own actions, her development toward speech took a normal course. However, as things improved, her difficulties became more pointed, and certain events, which were initially inexplicable, took on a new and remarkable significance.

Ahlem, of North African origin, was three years old when her mother first brought her to me. At nursery school, they were worried about her, for she never spoke, though she could understand some things, especially if spoken words were reinforced by appropriate gestures. The mother was expecting her second child, a boy, within a month, and she was also anxious to know whether he might be similarly affected. In our very first sessions, Ahlem was painfully shy, so withdrawn that she might not have been there at all. When I tried to make contact with her, she hid her eyes so as not to see me and held on to her mother. This active avoidance of me might actually be a good sign, although I soon realized that there was something else at work. She was scared, of course, but she also seemed to be completely helpless. For example, when I laid some colored pencils in her lap, in an attempt to encourage her to draw something, nothing happened. She did not knock them off her lap; she did not use them. She just sat there waiting, as though in a void, showing neither anxiety nor interest, without the slightest change of expression. Yet, as soon as I penciled a line on the paper, she was eager enough to do the same; she even initiated an exchange by handing me another pencil, so that I could do it again and she could copy. Her apathetic state was clearly not directed at me, as she was prepared to play at anything she could imitate. On the other hand, if I left it to her to initiate things, she went back to being dull, indifferent, as though switched off. That was all that happened at our first session, except that, when I said it was over and she understood more or less that it was time to go, she uttered a quiet little murmur, possibly expressing a feeling. So, though she was speechless and appeared not to understand words spoken to her, sounds she made did seem to convey meaning and affect.

Though it was clearly too early for me to have any reliable notions about what was wrong with the child, one or two possible ideas came to mind. On the one hand, her careful avoidance of any direct relating to me in the presence of her mother could be seen as a strategy for evading something she saw as a danger to be feared: she knew that, if she started to play with me, this would enable her mother to go away and be occupied with others, including possibly the baby soon to be born, and this was something she wanted to avoid at all costs. But, as well as that, there was her inability to initiate the slightest thing in play, which was at odds with the pleasure she took in imitating. So her obvious passivity was more than just a defense. The lack of organization observable in her manner suggested difficulties of a cognitive kind: it was as though when she was faced with the need to take an initiative, she was incapable of imagining, unable to think up the sequence of movements required to accomplish a program of action. In addition, there were manifest problems of an aphasiological kind. This had to be the explanation for why she never said anything despite the fact that, overall, language clearly had meaning for her, as she had shown by the sounds she uttered when told of the end of the first session. This was the tangle of causes making for the child's babylike passive resistance to the advent of a sibling who she feared would take her place.

Communication by Bodily Actions

By the time of the next session, there had been a change: when she caught sight of me in the waiting room, Ahlem came over and held out her hand. Once we were in the consulting room, she hid her eyes again, but I made this into the beginning of a game by imitating her gesture. Nevertheless, her mood was not good; soon she had had enough and pointed at her coat. It was clear not only that she wanted to leave but that she was perfectly able to use gestures to express what she meant. I told her I was aware that she wanted to leave and explained that it was too soon for her to do that. So she sat down again and agreed to do some drawing. We even contrived a second game: I drew circles on the board, inside each of which she put a dot, and these dots I said were "babies." That was all we did on that occasion, and our third encounter was not until after the summer vacation. As often happens after a longish interval, there had been another change: Ahlem still had nothing to say for herself, but she addressed me constantly through facial expressions and hand signals. For example, at one moment when I had drawn a little girl, she took a pencil and scribbled all over the mouth in the drawing, as though to prevent this rival from speaking. Her thinking and movements of affect were now communicable.

A Persistent Lack of Initiative

At the same time, as Ahlem became more active, some of her difficulties became more clearly visible. I was surprised, for instance, to see that certain objects of everyday use did not suggest any particular act to her: once, when she took a dolly onto her lap and I handed her a plate and a fork, expecting to see her start feeding the baby, she just held the utensils and did nothing. This reminded me of our very first encounter and her lack of response to the pencils: spontaneous action really was difficult for her; her only way of behaving was to take a cue from something done by someone else.

First Words

That was what explained the strangeness of the first words she spoke. Some months after we started work together, the child's mother told me with great pleasure that Ahlem had now begun to say words. However, her speech did not resemble the speech of other children: she read out numbers and the names of stations on the *métro*. This is a novel approach to language: a little girl who takes to reading before she can speak. However, it makes sense if one remembers that she had trouble with initiating action: in speaking, the problem must lie in how to initiate the actions required by phonation, without which the sounds of language cannot be produced. When she tries to produce these sounds, she can do so, as long as she has the support of the written forms associated with them, that is, numbers or letters. Gradually, she was to progress from reading written things to naming drawings and pictures; as soon as she had negotiated this hurdle, she was much more at ease with producing words and phonemes, and her speech started to develop in a more standard fashion. Before long it was present in the full range of its normal uses. For example, when we played "Memory," I would stop in the middle of dealing out the cards and ask, "More?" and she would nod and reply, "More!" Then, if she turned up a card with an apple on it matching the one in her hand, she would put them together and shout, "Other apple!" If she turned up the wrong card, she shook her head, showed her disappointment, and murmured "No" to herself. As soon as she knew how to pronounce something, she knew what it was for. Her use of language was varied: it was no longer just for naming or repeating; it underscored her inner life in all its diversity. In saying "Other apple!," for instance, she was bringing together two distinct points of thought: "apple," denoting the object, and "other," marking the effort of comparison that she had made and the recognition of the sameness of the two images. The process was under way, even though the phonetic quality of her longer utterances tended to suffer. Very soon she was also speaking during her games with dolls, commenting on the scenes she acted out: throwing a doll to the floor, she would say, "Fallen"; then, having picked it up and sat it back in its chair, she would say happily, "Not fallen." Language came to be linked with the pleasure of handling things, of making contrasts, of systematizing differences: "Same" and "Not same," like "Fallen" and "Not fallen," were woven into thought and action.

Disorder of Comprehension

By contrast, there were certain points where difficulties became quite marked and that seemed curious. In language, for example, though it soon became apparent that she did have some rudimentary syntax, which she used to tell me her baby had fallen, saying something that sounded like "Baby a' fallen" (rather than just using a simplified form such as "Baby fallen"), nonetheless, she had trouble understanding what was said to her. This would crop up in unexpected ways. One day when we had been playing with a chair belonging to a set of dolls' furniture and Ahlem was sitting on a child's chair, the end of the session arrived and I said, "Time to put the little chair away." I thought she would tidy away the toy chair, but she got up and pushed her own chair against the wall. For her, it was inconceivable that the words "little chair" could mean the toy, as though words had a single meaning, fixed once and for all, and as though she was incapable of modifying that meaning by reference to a context. Any mention of "chair" or "putting a chair away" was bound to be referring to the chair she had been sitting on, even though she knew that the little toy on which she had sat the doll was also called a chair. On the one hand there was knowledge, linked to the toy chair she could handle, and on the other there was linguistic awareness linked to her memory of the chair she was sitting on, but there was no association between the two. She could go from one to the other; but she could not fit the meaning of the word "chair" into the game, even though she was sitting there playing it with me, even though she could use the same word for chairs of different sorts, sizes, and shapes. If she heard me say the words "little chair," even while she was playing with the set of toy furniture, what she heard was of no use to her in locating, within the context of the game, the object I was speaking of. Her linguistic memories could summon up only a single situation. It was the same as with the pencils or the fork that I had given her: the image or the sound of a word tended to remain an empty thing for her; at best, they could mean something only inside the context of their initial appearance.

Tactile Exploration

Things could change only if she was able to start from a tactile exploration, as in the following example. In the waiting room one day, she was doing a jigsaw puzzle with her mother and appeared to be having trouble putting it together; though I was reluctant to interrupt her concentration on the problem, I did want her to finish it quickly so that we could go into the consulting room and start the session. So I tried to help her a little by taking hold of her right hand and running her middle finger around the edge of the piece she was trying to place. Having made her touch it and feel it, I showed her the gap where I thought she should fit it in. Unfortunately, being a pretty poor puzzler, I got it wrong and there was no fit. She, in a rather strange manner, tried my suggestion, found there was no fit, went calmly on with her exploration of the puzzle, and quite soon came upon the right gap. How was I to make sense of the effect that touch had had on her? As far as I could see, the sight of the shape of the piece conveyed nothing to her, no tactile sensation, whereas fingering the outline of the wooden shape enabled her eyes to "feel" and seek out among the ins and outs of the puzzle the place where it must fit. So it was active tactile exploration (which is very different from having a pencil or fork put into your inert hand) that helped Ahlem to mentally process and imagine slotting things among others without ever actually having done it. As soon as she handled an object, actively feeling it, it triggered something, and she could keep going. Some of her difficulties with speech also show the importance of this motor exploration and her awareness of movement: one day when she dropped a piece of the Russian doll set and it landed behind her chair, I said, by way of testing her comprehension, without pointing or looking at anything, "It fell behind your chair." She did not turn to look behind her; she just repeated, "Behind your chair" without understanding. But, as soon as she had spoken the words, her face brightened and she got up and looked for the missing object. For her, meaning came from her awareness of the actions of phonation needed to repeat the words. In the area of language, something happened that was comparable with what happened with the jigsaw: to see the meaning, she had to run her tongue around the edge of the phonemes. Unless she went through this intervening tactile and motor exploration, Ahlem could not transfer information from one level to another. All she could do was copy what she heard (that is, repeat) or superimpose one image on another, as long as they were identical. There were times when things were actually more complicated, when, even after a tactile exploration, her thinking was impeded by what she could see, as happened when we played a game called "Tactilo." This is a game in which each player has to feel little unseen wooden objects inside a bag and recognize on a display the images that correspond to them (there are small cubes, marbles, pyramids, cones, and cylinders). What happened was that when she abided by the rules and could not see the objects she was feeling, Ahlem was able to point at the right image, but when she cheated and looked at what she had in her hand, she became hesitant and got it wrong. The point is that the display shows the objects from a slightly unusual angle, and when she looked at what she had in her hand, she could not see it from exactly that angle. It was as though the sight of the object impeded her taking in what the tactile inspection told her and sent her off on a desperate attempt to superimpose two visual images on the same plane, the one on the display and the other that she tried to see by looking at the object. When her point of departure was an image or the sound of a word, she could manage identifications only of images that were identical. This was why, when looking at a picture book, she had trouble recognizing the same character in two separate frames if there was a slight difference in the character's position. The only way she could achieve a more stable representation was through tactile exploration and feel.

As time went on, however, the farther-reaching consequences of this difficulty were gradually mitigated by the development of a range of new aptitudes. Nowadays Ahlem can speak, though what she says is sometimes not very comprehensible. She takes the initiative in play, and her drawing gets better and better. Not long ago, she told me quite clearly that she wanted to see her very first drawings. When I opened the file for her, she sat for a moment gazing at her productions; then she pointed at one of them and said, "That one was with Mama and Laurent." It was clear that she had a perfect memory of the very first sessions when she used to come with her mother. These days she is alone in the consulting room with me, and we have come to share a whole sequence of rich experiences.

What I Learned from Working with Ahlem

In many respects, what happened with Ahlem was rather untypical of what happened with other children. For one thing, even today I would have trouble giving a reliable diagnosis based on her initial symptoms. It stands to reason that any idea of describing her disorder as autistic in nature or psychotic is ruled out by her solidly established ability to relate and by the richness of her nonverbal communication. From the very beginning, her way of responding to my exchange initiatives, though it was clumsy, was a definite indicator of her abilities in this area, as were the little sounds she made when I said the session was over and the fact that at our second session she pointed to her coat to show me she wanted to leave. There was certainly an element of dysphasia in her disorder. From the very first, it was clear that it was essentially a disorder of language, and a serious one at that. She spoke hardly at all, and she seemed also to have some difficulty in understanding things said to her. As is often the case at the outset of a course of therapy, there was so little verbal production that it was hard to tell whether I was confronted by a receptive disorder with effects on production (her inability to speak deriving from her inability to identify the sounds of the language) or solely an expressive disorder. There was also the fact of the child's bilingual background, the complicating effect of which was difficult to gauge. Even so, the seat of Ahlem's problems did not lie in these areas. She had other difficulties that belonged neither to communication nor to language. These were located in the register of nonlanguage cognition, a disorder that occurs in the area of the programming of motor activity (the project one must form before executing the simplest action) and, more specifically, in the programming of fine motor skills. The really striking thing about her was how difficult she found it to initiate any series of acts, to start putting into effect a plan of action. She looked as though no such idea could even occur to her, as though she could be set in motion only by someone else's suggestion. My own difficulty lay in trying to define the origin of this inability to program appropriate acts. The hypothesis that attracted me was this: prima facie, Ahlem seemed unable to link up information she received from different sources and to modulate it according to context. What she could see did not relate either to any memory she might have retained about what had just happened in our exchange or in a game or to any of the more general information held in her long-term memory, particularly in the register of language. There was some sort of cognitive dissociation that prevented her from programming, thinking, and communicating. What gave me this idea was the two episodes with the jigsaw puzzle and the little chair. In order to put a piece of jigsaw into the puzzle, one must be able to imagine how it will fit among the other pieces already in place, which Ahlem could not do until I made her finger the outline of the piece she was holding. Had I not helped her in this way, the image of the shape would have remained irrelevant to her and would not have helped her formulate a course of action. She did not transfer the visual into the tactile, though for her it was apparently the tactile that set in motion the assembly plan that could then guide her hand in the sequential activity of puzzling. This same hypothesis of dissociation helped me understand the episode with the little chair. When I said it was time to put the little chair away, the only conceivable meaning that the words "little chair" could have for her was as a reference to the smallest of the real chairs standing around the table, and not to the toy chair that she was playing with. She could not alter the reference of the term in accordance with her present situation. The source of this misunderstanding was that the words used were inextricably bound to the single context of chairs that people can sit on. She could not associate the words I spoke with our actual context, in which there were little chairs that dolls but not people could sit on.

I suspect it was this cognitive difficulty that was peculiar to Ahlem. It did, of course, have an effect on her communication, which it considerably inhibited, at least at the beginning. It also had an effect on her language and reinforced some aspects of her dysphasia. Nonetheless, this cognitive peculiarity was not in itself either a disorder of communication or a disorder of language. And the identification of it as a specifically different disorder substantially clarified the picture given by the general symptomatology.

Nowadays, Ahlem is a little girl who enjoys life. She still requires treatment from a speech therapist, and I continue to see her regularly. However, my work with her has turned into very straightforward psychotherapy. She does drawings and talks to me about her everyday life and anything she finds bothersome in her relationships or within the family circle. This treatment, too, should soon come to an end. She even said to me recently, "I really like coming here to see you. But can you tell me why I'm still coming?"

7

Lanny, or the Silence of the Mad Child

René Diatkine was fond of saying, "The worst may not happen." Sometimes, even though a successful outcome seems unlikely, when there are
obvious signs that a course of treatment may be discontinuous or irregular or may even be aborted, something nevertheless can be achieved as
long as the therapist is aware of these untoward possibilities. This was
what happened with Lanny.

When I first encountered Lanny, a little African boy of three and a
half, he ran all over the place yelling but never spoke a word. The impression one had of him was that here was a child who was insane. His
family had been in France for four years, five of them living in a single
room rented from an Asian restaurant owner who threatened to cut off
the electricity if their money ran out. Lanny was the one worst affected:
his twin brother and a little sister were doing relatively well, but he was
strange. When he was not in a state of agitation, he would stand for hours
at the window, now and again laughing to himself for no apparent reason, in a void, not attending to anything. I gradually came to realize that
his father believed the child was under a curse, an idea that had no substance for me until the day when he told me what Lanny's madness meant
within his own life story. I learned this on meeting them again after the
family had disappeared for two months. Nevertheless, curiously enough,
Lanny's treatment was exemplary, though the regularity of his psychic
progress was at great variance with the irregularity of his visits. There were
times when he stopped coming, because the family was out of contact
with me; there were other times when he was so agitated that the whole
thing seemed fruitless. Despite all this, we did make progress: a readiness

to take advantage of chance and the child's spontaneous initiatives now and then produced sudden advances, which, seen in hindsight, form a regular pattern. It was almost as though Lanny had been fast-forwarded through the initial stages of a normal child's symbolic development. First, there was the establishment of exchange and nonverbal communication, followed by onomatopoeic utterances associated with play. Then he gave evidence of having acquired several set expressions. Because of this improvement, the essential elements of his disorder became more visible: in most areas, Lanny was very skilled in the reproduction of actions he could witness but very unskilled when it came to imagining them spontaneously.

My first encounter with this child left me with mixed feelings. His general behavior, as I had expected, was affected by constant swinging between prostration and agitation. With the aim of calming him, I made a point of moving as little as possible and never addressing him directly. First contact was achieved when I placed a set of Russian dolls in front of him and started to take them apart. This seemed to interest him: he took up the tops of them, turned them over, and sniffed inside them, intrigued no doubt by the smell of pine and varnish. Then he made a clumsy attempt to stand the smaller ones on top of the larger ones, like hats. Something in this struck me at once: one of the top pieces having dropped to the floor, I reached down for it and put it back on the table, and Lanny, a few moments later, also stooped down to get the hat that I had already retrieved. It looked as though he remembered that something had fallen but had not paid attention to my action. The point was not that he had not seen me do it: it was that what he saw was irrelevant while he was engrossed in something else. His thoughts, preoccupations, and action did not function in response to his perceptions of the outside world, because when he was immersed in something, anything that he could see remained extraneous, meant nothing to him, evoked no response. This, however, was not invariable, and there were moments when he was aware of his surroundings. A little later, when we started to draw, he paid attention to what I was doing. He was interested in the markers, took them unprompted, and drew concentric circles and parallel lines. I was struck by the clear superiority of his graphic aptitudes over his other abilities. As a way of establishing communication with him, I started to copy each of the lines he drew; before I made each of my marks on the board, I whispered, "Again?" This was also a way of making sure that he was in agreement with me, that we were doing something together, and that he was the one in charge. To begin with, he gave no sign of anything, but his role as initiator gradually grew until I eventually heard him repeating "Again" after me in a barely audible voice. For the moment, this repetition was not quite real speech: it was just a way of doing what I was doing, the beginnings of a turn-taking game. As such, it showed an interest in exchange but did not amount to a true signifier. Imperceptibly, though, it became a sign of his acquiescence to the suggestion that I should copy his lines.

After this first encounter, my feeling was that, though the child was given to extreme agitation and became easily disorganized, this did not rule out possible contact with him. As we had seen, for example, with the markers, communication had been achieved. Speech had been minimal, but his murmurings in response to me, barely perceptible though they were, showed that he could think of sounds you can make with your mouth as objects of exchange. Not long afterward, I noticed, too, that he really did engage with another person's spoken word: he listened to what was said to him and tried to do what was asked of him, albeit with surprising clumsiness at times. In this connection, a remarkable thing happened one day when he was playing with a box, enjoying opening and closing it. The lid got stuck, and, seeing the difficulty he had in opening it, I encouraged him by saying, "Open." As soon as he heard this, he stopped what he was doing, got up, and went to the door of my consulting room, as though I had said, "Open the door." He had interpreted my word as an order and had gone to comply with it. He had actually understood the word "Open" but without being able to extract it from the frame in which he was probably used to hearing it: for him, "Open" applied to doors, which, in his inability to either abstract the word from the situation where it belonged or transpose its sense to another situation, was the context he was looking for when he went toward the door. Even when the other situation was clearly marked by our shared interest and though we had been playing together at opening and closing the box, it made no difference: "opening" and "closing" were things that could be done only with doors. Unlike what I had noted with the Russian dolls, his difficulty here had nothing to do with not perceiving things but meant that he had not managed to decontextualize them, as we say. The word spoken meant a particular motion to be gone through with a single kind of object: in his mind, opening a door by pulling the handle downward, opening a box by removing its lid, and opening a tap by turning it on were such different actions, done in such different contexts, that they could not possibly entail doing the same thing. Metaphorical assimilation, which enables us to see a sameness in things that remain different in other respects, was impossible. So, on hearing the word "open," Lanny was incapable of starting from the meaning common to all the different ways of opening things and of finding a use for the word in his present situation. A similar thing happened on another occasion when I said "Look" to attract his attention to a drawing of a man: he got up and went to the window, which to him was the only conceivable place where an order to look could be carried out.

This inability to separate words from their familiar context so as to relate them to the present situation and to intended meanings different from the usual ones is found in other children. Though most such children also have serious difficulties with language, I do not consider this particular trouble to be of itself a linguistic disorder. I see it as an effect that a nonlanguage disorder can have on language; I have already discussed this problem in connection with Ahlem.

That said, what diagnosis could one arrive at in the case of Lanny? The boy manifestly presented severe autistic features, and the least that could be said was that nonverbal exchange with him was far from easy. For all that, he did not live in a world of his own. Unlike some autistic children, he was not a prisoner of stereotyped behaviors, utterly indifferent to anything outside himself. He was interested by my way of imitating him, and on occasion he would join in a turn-taking game. He even came to be the one directing my imitation of the circles that he drew on the board. Also, even though he mistook the meaning of what I said to him, he heard something in my words that had meaning for him, something he tried to understand and act upon. A psychoanalytical diagnosis of the child's disorder would have to classify it under childhood psychosis. Childhood psychosis differs from autism in two respects: on the one hand, there is the ability to relate to others, though it may be greatly impaired; on the other, the child is not totally absorbed in the pleasure afforded by his own sensations or his repetition of a single action. This was certainly the case with Lanny: he maintained a link with me and in addition was able, with a little assistance, to avail himself of mental representations to alter something in what he did. For example, even though he was greatly taken with the piny, varnishy smell of the Russian dolls and sniffed them before starting to fit them together, he was capable of going beyond that. With a little help and encouragement, he would try putting them inside or on top of one another. What these manipulations showed was that he was in fact capable of using representation in connection with objects that he discovered. His communication was much more impaired than Ahlem's. But, like her, he presented a particular nonlanguage disorder of cognition that manifested itself in the fact that spontaneous motor projects were foreign to him. So he could not properly make up games or drawings, unless he had been given a pattern to follow. As with Ahlem, the best hypothesis seemed to be that his disorder derived from a disjunction among his sources of information. It may well be that the progress made with him came about because the continuing contact with me eventually enabled the disjunction to be replaced by connections and links that then fostered the development of nonverbal communication and his subsequent access to speech.

Two months after the beginning of treatment, I had seen Lanny only seven times, not quite once a week. His language was still virtually non-existent, though his nonverbal communication and his aptitudes for exchange were much improved, and he had become more expressive: seeing me come into the waiting room, he would smile, rather than drift away into his systematic vacancy. He was also the initiator in play and was not content to merely copy me, going straight to the board, for example, doing a squiggle, then handing me the pad so that I could erase it. A more recent ritual that we had developed was the following: as my consulting times were always fixed for after-school hours, when it was beginning to get dark, and as he seemed to be attracted by the street lights, we stood at the window watching for cars. I dramatized this with a series of short utterances, punctuating the appearance and disappearance of cars: "Look out. Another one. There it goes. Gone." At first, Lanny just repeated my little statements in an undertone as he pointed to the cars I drew attention to. However, after a while, each time he saw a vehicle coming into his field of vision, he started to accompany his pointing with a sound like "cr," which could be an attempt at *encore* (= "again," "another"). He even invented other hide-and-seek type games, such as showing me the end of a ruler then concealing it under a piece of paper. I was reasonably satisfied with the way things were turning out.

Unfortunately, the family moved to the outer suburbs, leaving an address that was incomplete. It took two months and some cross-checking by the team's social worker to track them down. When she spoke to the father, he eventually agreed to talk to us, but without Lanny. He had something he wanted to say; during the talk we had with him, he told us straight out that there was something wrong with his son: he would stand at the window, staring at nothing, wholly absorbed in himself, muttering incomprehensible words, then would burst out laughing without rhyme or reason, and the father would always have to interrupt him and bring him back to reality. This description of the child's behavior struck me: though the father had not expressed it in so many words, I had the impression that he believed his son was subject to intermittent madness. This called to mind all those other parents who, in similar circumstances, would say: "My child's not insane, he's just a bit dreamy, he likes playing by himself. He's still a bit of a baby, but I'm sure things will sort themselves out in time," by which they mean it is "others" (the school, the doctor, a grandparent, other children's parents) who keep saying there is a problem, whereas they know better. But, for Lanny's father, the child was not just a little retarded: there were times when he was crazy. Once I had grasped this, I asked him whether he had ever come across other children like his son. He did not give a direct answer but told me that, after he had left his village to come to France, there had been cases, and he went straight on to tell me a different story, about his own father, who had also had a bout of madness many years before, one night when he had decided to sleep outside his hut and two giants had appeared in the darkness, though no one else could see them. One of them, an evil spirit without a head, was out to harm him, while the other was trying to protect him. As he was a good Muslim, the good spirit had defeated the headless giant, and the grandfather saved his reason. In the giants, twins like Lanny and his brother, one of them good and the other having lost his head, there was a clear symbolic logic that I kept to myself. Lanny's father then told me about a serious accident that had happened to the child when he was just under a year old; when I pressed him to say more about the circumstances, he closed up and said everything was already "in the file." I asked him whether he thought Lanny, like the grandfather, had come across two invisible giants, one good and the other evil. My idea was that, since Lanny's twin had the Muslim forename Ali, it must have been he who had been spared by the good spirit, while Lanny had lost his head because of the other one; this the father accepted. I told him I could do nothing without the assistance of both parents. After some thought, the father said, "Okay, I can come with Lanny and my wife, though it's a long way from our new home." As he took his leave of the social worker and me, he called both of us by our names, a sign of his recognition of us, a hint that things were returning to normal. When he had gone, it occurred to us that Lanny's parents were a "reconstituted" couple: each of them had had a childless first marriage; soon after coming together, they had had their twins. Lanny's misfortunes could also be seen as the result of a curse put on them by the rejected partners. The meaning one gives to calamity is not a "cause" of it, but it can contribute to the way it becomes set in the mind, because then "the worst must happen."

As arranged, the whole family turned up for the following session. The father was in charge of things, and, of course, as soon as he started to do anything, Lanny took refuge in disorganized agitation, running to the window, climbing onto his mother's lap, and was soon out of control. I said, "Well, Lanny is more than a match for us all," with which the father agreed, reassured to see that I was as incompetent with his son as he was. Things settled down, and a game was organized: the father pointed to each of us in turn, and Lanny pushed his toy car toward the one indicated. When I thought the game had gone on long enough, I decided to complicate it: when the car was pushed toward me, I took it and hid it under the lid of a box. Unfortunately and unexpectedly, Lanny did not point at the lid as a way of asking me for the car. He ran at me, jerked the lid roughly aside, and took the car. My attempt was therefore a partial failure, since the child had chosen to put a quick end to it. But it was also partly successful, since he had done it without an outburst, without running around in all directions, and since he came straight back into the game and went on pushing the car.

Lanny's relation to what he could not see was therefore very complex: he was unable to point at the car when it was hidden, as though unsure of its continued existence (and what that represented for him); even so, since he fetched it out again, he did know that the car was still there, and he could keep his mind on it.

This manifestation of the child's partial responsiveness and ability to acquire skills encouraged me to try something else. I shaped a tunnel from a sheet of paper and stood it on the table. Then I showed Lanny how we could run the car through and have it reappear at the other end. This time, the game worked: the car's disappearance inside the tunnel was temporary, and, since it reappeared of its own accord at the other end, he could cope with the complication I had introduced. He actually found it amusing. The visible/invisible/visible sequence lent itself to integration in his procedures. Perhaps it also reminded him a little of his own game with the ruler when he made it appear then disappear under a piece of paper.

A little later in this same session, Lanny himself spontaneously introduced a new development. He took a gray elephant and a rag doll with gray hair and held them close to my shirt, which also happened to be gray that day. Next, he took a second elephant out of the box, with its baby, and made them walk through the paper tunnel, in single file. The social worker, who was also present at this family session, said, "The baby, too," by way of a comment on the presence of the little elephant behind the two big ones. As though this remark were an interpretation cutting to the quick of his psyche, Lanny immediately left the three elephants (gray, like my shirt) and went to stare at two ashtrays standing on the desk. There were two of them, like the couple of elephant parents, but, unlike elephants, ashtrays do not have babies. Here, there is a symbolic link that can be made sense of. Lanny's sequence of little scenes: the way he made the elephants walk through the tunnel, then the way he turned away from them to refocus on the pair of ashtrays, are evidence of a psychic movement comparable to those that can be observed in young children who are normal, with its displacements and its repetitions. The elephant couple going under the bridge with their baby was undoubtedly the beginning of a symbolic game. The social worker's comment must have been an acute crystallization of something in the child's mind, making him give up his first dramatization of it and begin again with a different couple (the ashtrays) who were safer than the elephants because they could not have babies.

As this sequence shows, Lanny seemed to have developed a particular symbolic aptitude. He was capable of metaphor, displacement, and association. Because metaphor usually requires language, we tend to think of it as growing out of experience of speech. This case, however, seems to me to show that there is a infraverbal stage of metaphor, which works as a kind of prerequisite for linguistic expression. A similar thing had already happened with him more than once. For example, during an earlier session I was gently teasing him by taking away a car he was playing with. To make him come and ask for it back, I kept it in my hand in a way that let him see some of it. He, no doubt wishing I would hand it over, went behind me and covered one of the lenses of my glasses with one of his hands, as though to say, "Stop half-hiding the car in your hand and give it back." As on the other occasion with the elephants, there was a metaphorical element in the game; unlike the other occasion, the metaphorical element was a real sign: Lanny covered up only one of my eyes, not both of them, telling me via metaphor that I was partly hiding what he wanted. In so doing, he also imposed on me a privation comparable with the one I had imposed on him. Some time later, he came back to this hide/show game, using an ashtray with a retractable base.

It was no doubt this new aptitude for play and displacement that improved Lanny's ability to put up with frustration. In any case, his behavior changed. When I announced the end of the session, he was now capable of tidying things, instead of running around throwing things as he had done in the early days. This was a development that his nursery school confirmed: at the beginning of the year, he had stood away from the others, alternating bouts of yelling with moments of withdrawal, whereas now he could fit into group activities and say "Me" when he wanted to take his turn. In speech, too, he seemed to have made progress: rather than acting out his opposition, he now spoke it and was able to say "No." He was able to say when something was not right: one day, when I put a pillow under a doll's head, he took it away, saying, "No good." When there was insufficient space on a table to lay out pictures, I heard him murmur, "There's no more room." Speech enabled him to crystallize the disparity between what he wanted and what he could see. Similarly, in his scenarios and games, he gave orders to his characters and made them speak. Reappearances were welcomed with "Peekaboo!" and disappearances with "Bye-bye." When he sat a bus driver down at the steering wheel, he said, "Sit in your seat," possibly something he had heard at school. What most struck me was that he could now use words in different contexts, whereas not long before, statements like "Open" and "Look" referred solely to something done with a door or at a window. In social things, too, he was capable of replying with full statements properly placed, such as "I'm staying in the lunch room," "I'm staying for a snack," or "Mama's coming to get me." And when he played "Memory," he could put names to the pictures on the cards as he turned them up. He also knew by heart a great number of nursery rhymes and loved to repeat them. Written language was another area of achievement: he was very interested in books; as long as he was dealing with standard letters and shapes, he displayed great skill. He could write his own name and his brother's in block letters; and if he saw the word *camion* (= "truck"), say, he could point at the truck in the toybox. Of course, none of this meant that his speech was properly grounded. In fact, the more he consolidated his most primary level of speech and nonverbal communication, becoming bolder and more inventive in expression, the clearer it became that he had difficulty in remembering the proper shapes of words. Whenever there was nothing to help him, something he had just heard, for instance, or a written word, a picture, or an act required by a social situation (such as a handshake, meaning that one says "Hello"), the shapes of words were beyond his grasp. This meant that his language turned into an unbroken singsong babble of barely recognizable sounds, though the intonation was good. In other words, given that his preverbal communication had stabilized and that verbal communication was beginning to take shape, his particular mode of dysphasia became more apparent: his was a receptive disorder. He would need more time before any significant improvement could be observed. Spontaneous actions or gestures, of whatever sort, were still delicate operations for him: he needed a model to copy, some kind of support, whether it was a matter of knowing the movements of phonation required to produce a word, a graphic gesture needed to draw something, or a sequence mimed in a game.

Nevertheless, despite these undoubted drawbacks, Lanny eventually acquired the ability to construct a story, which, in my view, involves the most advanced and delicate use of language. As will be seen, he did not reach this stage until he had come to terms with an unexpected traumatic event that helped him realize not only that he could think unaccompanied but that he had to. Unaccompanied thinking meant thinking without my being able to understand him.

Therapeutic relationships established with children produce bonds that are so intense that for a long time the therapist's presence and attention are crucial to any progress a child may make: a child who feels misunderstood by the therapist, or at a loss if the therapist is absent, may be completely helpless, and one can have the impression that things are falling apart. It is a great step forward for a child, when help is required for overcoming a difficulty, to be able to depend on someone other than the therapist. As will be seen, this was what happened with Lanny during a session when I had been particularly unreceptive. A third person was present: since sessions with the child had become more and more irregular and the family had stopped attending them, his father had eventually agreed to Lanny's being accompanied to and from my consulting room by someone else, and a young woman specializing in linguistics, who was helping me study the boy's linguistic progress, had undertaken to do this. She attended the sessions, then took him home. On this particular day, Lanny would not be satisfied until I had drawn him a house with smoke coming out of the chimney. The trouble was that I had drawn my smoke in a closed shape, like a cloud, and not in the form he wanted, that of a spiral, such as one might draw for the smoke from a man's pipe, for example. There was something wrong with my smoke, and I could not understand what it was. It was my young colleague who realized why Lanny was so irritated and who pointed out how the smoke should be redrawn in a way that would satisfy him. As soon as I had made the appropriate changes to the drawing, he showed his satisfaction and copied my spiral of smoke, after which he added his name, as though the fact of having been at last understood had helped him recover the contours of his identity. My lack of understanding had led him to the painful discovery of his individuation. Because of the support of the young woman, he had coped with this experience without needing to withdraw into anxiety or get worked up as he used to. Her understanding him had enabled him to put up with the knowledge that he and I were not in complete harmony with each other. What this had done for him was reveal that his psychic space was separate from mine and that he could thereby find support in someone else. He had become aware of a state intermediate between absolute oneness and the agitation (or depression) brought on by emotional distress. From her support he had drawn the realization that he could make me accept him in his difference from me, even though I had not been agreeable to this at first. Thanks to her, he had been through a momentary abandonment on my part, followed by a reunion. By the time of the next session, there was a change in his language. First, he recapitulated the spiral of smoke episode, making plain the importance it had for him and ensuring that we were now as one on that matter. Then, spontaneously, he started to recount what had happened at a party held at his nursery school. This was something, an event where I had not been present, that he could now tell me about, since he knew I was capable of understanding things that I had not experienced with him. When a child reaches the stage of talking to me about things that neither of us can see and that he is the only one to have experience of, my impression is that, however faulty his language, he has achieved mastery of all its uses.

I look on Lanny as a case from which many lessons can be learned. For one thing, it led to one of those very favorable outcomes that therapists like to see as proof of their own brilliance, even though there are plenty of other cases that advise against such presumptuousness. On the face of things, everything seemed to make such an outcome implausible: the severity of his initial disorder, the undeniable element of autism in the pathology, and the problems that arose during treatment (moving house and the temporary disappearance of the family, in particular). Despite all of this, something happened to make this child improve much more markedly than other children whose initial disorders seemed no less severe than his. In retrospect, one wishes there could be some surety about what it was that worked, which of the signs, if only I had noticed them at the outset, might have presaged such a positive final outcome. With hindsight, I think I can isolate two factors: one of them was how the boy was able to accept my offers to play, and the other was the interest he took in what I said to him. Both of these factors actually indicate the same thing: a degree of responsiveness toward others, despite the obstacles to communication. And if it is possible to see a disorder of communication as definitely resulting from an impairment, rather than as a conscious and intended avoidance, there is another ground for hope. With this child, my suspicion that the disorder derived from cognitive dissociation arose quite early on, and that I believe was the disorder that, as our exchanges proceeded, underwent some improvement. I must admit, however, that in most cases, such predictive insights occur to me only afterward.

8

Louis, or Shared Monologue

A Strange Entry into Language

Louis was a boy of five, devoid of language. As a result of the combined efforts of several therapists, he managed to come to language. The most striking thing about this was the way he did it. In general, when a child starts to speak, his first words serve to convey his surprise and his desires and to make known his demands. With Louis, however, things were different. Initially, his language was a single long monologue, saying nothing about his desires but describing whatever he could see in front of him or things and events that this reminded him of. It was as though words could come to him only when he was in the presence of things, as though language could never be anything but a game played in solitude, divorced from exchange and communication. Curiously enough, it was through simulation and narration that he gradually developed the ability to use language to ask something of me.

Permeability in Person

The first time he came to see me, I was struck at once by his manner, which was very self-effacing and reminded me of Ahlem. However, un-like her, it would not have been right to say he withdrew from contact. Nor did he appear to have any particular difficulty in matching appropriate actions to a situation. Face to face, the impression he gave was of being totally insubstantial. In any exchange, he very soon faded away and took on a sort of transparency. His preschool teacher said, "When he arrived, he was slumped on his father's back and his father was holding him on with one arm, like a shapeless lump of something." That was an image of Louis that stayed in my mind for a long time, as did the inertness of his hand and the indefinite feel of it in mine as we greeted each other, or the way his eyes looked through me when I approached him in the waiting room. His eyesight was very bad, so he wore huge glasses, which were always askew on his nose, so I imagined he must have trouble making out the face of anyone he talked to and was unable to infer what another person was feeling. This would mean that he was never sure of being understood, and it might explain his tendency to withdraw, which might be responsible for the fact that his language could never get past the monologue stage. There was also the fact that he could speak only of things that were there in front of him, which ruled out any expression of desire.

For a long time, there was something strange about my dealings with Louis, strange though not difficult. In fact, from the very first session, we established a relationship through play: in the toybox, he found a piece of fence in soft plastic, which he folded over and stood on the table in front of us; I did the same with another piece, which I set down beside his. Then, without a word, I held out my hand for him to give me a third piece, and this he did. My imitation of his spontaneous activity brought about a sharing of interest, from which exchange followed. He paid attention to my action (helped no doubt by the holding out of a hand, which was more explicit than a facial expression would have been); he understood it and responded. A few moments later, he took the box onto his knees, and I made a piglet jump into it, which made him smile, though without looking at me. By the end of the session, although I knew he was open to turn-taking games, I did not know whether he was capable of spontaneously drawing my attention to something or pointing at things or whether it might ever occur to him that he could make me share what he was thinking. Nor had I yet heard the sound of his voice, not having even attempted anything in that line. What seemed of immense importance to me was that he could meet an adult who was willing to share an exchange with him without forcing him to speak.

The Two Registers of Speech

Fortunately, Louis's silence did not last long. For one thing, in our games of exchanging objects, he very quickly started to repeat in a whisper the few things I said, underlining our alternation of action with an alternation of speech. For another, in addition to this whispering, which was restricted to our face-to-face exchanges, he showed me another way of speaking that he had. This consisted of a loud voice, almost pedantic, sounding rather like the didactic tone a concerned parent might use to a child; and he soon took to using it for talking about our shared themes, in particular his drawings. Unfortunately, however, the words he spoke were usually incomprehensible. So, by way of acknowledgment of his efforts, while not trying to conceal my uncertainty, I just repeated in an interrogative intonation the sounds I thought he was making.

Crisis and Language

From the point of view of language, it was an emergency that brought about real change. This happened on the first occasion when we had a session without his parents. Having come with me to the consulting room, he did not understand until we had gone in that they were to stay outside; when he realized this, he started to run from one side of the room to the other, trying as hard as he could to open the door and escape. It was at that moment, faced with the closed door and still in great agitation, that I heard him say quite distinctly, *Fermé porte, clé !* (= "Shut door, lock!"). It sounded not like a statement in three parts but like three consecutive statements, blurted out in the stress of the situation. It struck me as curious that this stress should have resulted in language, rather than in massive disorganization, and I wondered under what conditions an emotional emergency of this order would require such a qualitative leap. I continue to wonder about the role of this violent blockage in the emergence of Louis's first genuine language, and I am still struck by the fact that what he said, "Shut door, lock," was not a request (such as, say, "Open door") but rather a kind of observation spoken to himself and not to me, unaccompanied by so much as a glance in my direction.

Since Freud, we know about the link between frustration, absence, and the emergence of thought. We know that the thought of something, our representation of it, is not a copy made in its presence but a sort of processed hallucination, the function of which is to calm the tension caused by the lack of the thing itself. Under ordinary circumstances, neither thought nor words with their associated symbols come to mind to express what we see. They are not linked to the present: their role is to console for absence. If we accept that speech arises out of a lack of satisfaction, this may explain why Louis started to speak properly at a moment when things were not as he wished. That, however, is insufficient as an explanation, for in that case he should have asked something of me. Yet, what he did say was not a request of any sort: it was an exclamation, not the expression of a wish, and, most importantly, it was not addressed to me. His utterance sounded as though its sole function was to enable the boy in his panic to identify and define the cause of what was upsetting him. Once this was done, he could rid himself of his emotional disturbance by expelling the words that characterized it, as though the air he exhaled through speech freed him from all the representations linked to the signifiers he spoke, as though this was a way of letting out the thing that hurt, which for him was associated with the words "Shut door, lock." So, instead of using the spoken word to evoke and manipulate the representation of a thing that was missing, what he was trying to do was remove the pain of the real by expelling the words that defined the real. Emotional disturbance gave vent to genuine language, though it was still language unaddressed to anyone else, a monologue expressive only of his effort to define the source of his pain and let it out. What was peculiar to Louis was not so much this use of monologue, which is no more than one can hear in anyone's exclamation of pained surprise, but the fact that he had no other usage. Devoid as he was of any adequate link to other people, whatever he said was self-addressed. And, since his only starting point was what he could see, there was no way he could speak in advance about anything he might wish. All he could do through language was say what was upsetting him, and that was what was expressed in "Shut door, lock."

Despite its shortcomings, this leap into language proper had repercussions on the child's two ways of speaking, affecting both his whispered language and his loud, pedantic voice. Initially, repeating my words in an undertone when we were face to face had been nothing more than his way of accommodating to a turn-taking game. However, it gradually became a way of taking over the meaning of my words by saying them himself. Also, he gradually borrowed some of my words, such as "again" and "also," and used them unprompted in play. As for the loud voice, its register also evolved. In addition to the comments he already made on his drawings, he now started to comment on things outside the window. Whenever I pointed at something that seemed to interest him (rain falling, umbrellas, cars passing), or if I announced possible changes to the street scene (appearances or disappearances of certain umbrellas or cars), he would start to speak in his pedantic voice. Sometimes he would put words to this scene, and sometimes it was a starting point for mentioning other things of the same name, many different umbrellas, for instance, those carried by passersby, but also his own umbrella or the one owned by "Aunty Christiane" (his preschool teacher, who had gone away). Strictly speaking, such statements were not descriptions but more a way of making it manifest that a word such as "umbrella," for instance, could be applied in different contexts (the street, the room, memory), reminiscent of how a child will come upon a picture of a telephone in a book, then turn to point at the telephone near the door behind him.

Later, with the benefit of our joint attention, Louis broadened the register of this loud voice and used it to express thoughts and preoccupations suggested by what was happening in his presence.

Metaphor and Thinking beyond the Self

Even so, for a long time, Louis's way of naming things went on being bothersome. When he was playing with a plastic Playmobil baby, for instance, he called it a "tortoise," probably because of the gored bonnet it had on its head, and a dry sponge he called "bread," because it was full of small holes and reminiscent of a slice of coarse loaf. It was not that he mistook the baby for a tortoise or the dry sponge for bread: the words were metaphors, analogous to those one can observe in the linguistic development of normal children going through the stage when they come out with their made-up words. However, unlike such children, Louis clung to his way of naming things and would not change. This was not to be explained by any stubbornness. It was as though, in his view, the small holes in the dry sponge—the very feature that made him call it "bread"— were the only thing that could stand for the sponge. A sponge, of course, to the mind of anyone able to think freely about it, may have associations with a slice of bread, because of its consistency, or with a bar of soap, because of its shape, or even with a damp cloth, because of the use it is put to. If a representation is to be properly and fully available, all the details that inhere in it must be equally able to stand for it in its entirety, and one must be capable of varying the relevant aspect of it depending on what one means. In other words, one must be able to think beyond the self. It was precisely this that Louis was incapable of doing: he was stuck on the one detail that struck him, could not move it to the background, and clung to the word that had that meaning for him. This cognitive inflexibility was apparent elsewhere, too, notably in the fact that he was often bothered by different representations of the same object, for example, an open umbrella and a closed umbrella, which made him hesitate to use the one word for them. His trouble with thinking outside himself could be seen too in his way of organizing the representation of an object. For example, in any object, the thing he saw as a point or frame of reference could not itself be seen in reference to anything else, so that, if he was doing a picture of a car, say, he would draw the outline of the bodywork in a single continuous stroke, taking care to include the wheel arches, but the wheels themselves were nowhere to be seen. For him, the wheels were unimaginable. The point was that, in his representation of a car, it was the bodywork that was the frame and point of reference: it contained inside it everything that could be imagined, the engine, the steering wheel, even the driver and the passengers. There is, of course, one thing that stands outside this frame, and that is the wheels. Therein lies the problem: by being outside, the wheels are extraneous to the frame of reference supplied by the bodywork. As the bodywork is supported by the wheels, it is the wheels that offset it. In order to include a car's wheels in a drawing, one has to think from a perspective outside one's own, stop seeing the bodywork as the sole point of reference for the whole, and see the wheels as a new point of reference enabling one to plot the position of the earlier one in relation to it. By putting in the indents for the wheels while leaving out the wheels themselves, Louis was evading this need to think outwardly and diversely. It was a procedure that brought to mind another child who drew an island and told me he felt like putting the sea inside it instead of all around, even though he was perfectly well aware that islands are surrounded by water. Just like Louis's bodywork, the outline of the island represented an all-inclusive frame that should contain all the elements involved, including the sea.

Communication plus Eclipses

After eighteen months of work, and despite the persistence of some difficulties, Louis's communication had become stronger, though his moments of being absent while present, as well as his sudden incongruities of speech, had not entirely disappeared. For our link to remain stable, I had to be the constant mirror and guarantor of his wishes and intents: if I stopped doing this, he would forget what he wanted and lose the thread of whatever exchange we were engaged in. When this happened, I did not usually realize it until afterward. It happened, for instance, in our games of hide-and-seek: to begin with, everything seemed to suggest that he knew the point of the game, since he would respond to my "Peekaboo"; so I hid behind a pillar, stuck my head out to say "Peekaboo," and pulled it in again. However, Louis's grasp of the game was tenuous, and he was not really engaged in it: when I said, "Peekaboo," he would repeat it, but without making any move to go and find me once I was hidden. He did not see my saying "Peekaboo" as a signal for him to get ready to look for me. He repeated it after me, but then lost touch with the meaning of the game. In order for him to play and see a meaning in it, he needed me to be looking at him and thus assuring him of the permanence of his own image. I had to be the depositary of what he wanted and what he felt; as soon as I stepped out of that role, he lost all his consistency and outline. This was what happened if I hid from him, but also if he had to assert himself against me: when I would conceal an object that he was playing with, he was incapable of coming over and taking it away from me, which was what many other children would have done. He just gave up and seemed to forget what it was he wanted. Without my support, his purposes petered out.

Uneven Development of Language

I am now going to tell how Louis's language came to make its final change. This was about two years after the beginning of treatment, a time when the general format of our sessions was well established and the sequence of activities regular. We would start by sitting for a moment at a table outside the consulting room, blowing on a plastic beaker to make it roll around. Next we would go in, and Louis would roll "balls" of plasticine from bits of it that he pulled off a lump held in my hand; then he placed the balls inside a toy wardrobe. Sometimes I would roll one of the balls into a "snake." After that, we would stand at the window so that Louis could comment on what was to be seen. It was generally at that moment, if not while he was making the balls of plasticine, that he would talk about what he had been doing elsewhere, at school, perhaps, or with his father.

Louis was therefore capable of sharing with me an activity with plasticine, although this cooperation gave rise to no direct exchange. What he put into words at that point was memories: for example, because of the balls of plasticine, he would tell me that, before each of our sessions, he went to the "toilets" with his father; the street scenes brought to mind associations with school. However, apart from that, he was still unable to address a direct request to me: if I took hold of something that he wanted, he could not say, "Give me." This I found intriguing, for might one not think, prima facie, that to put a past situation into words requires a far greater degree of linguistic maturity than to formulate a request arising out of a present exchange? Nevertheless, that was the case with Louis: he could speak of what he was feeling and of what he had seen, but he could not ask me to do anything. What was particularly surprising here was that, despite this, he was perfectly capable of playing his part in turn-taking games. The hypothesis I eventually formed to explain this peculiar state of affairs was that, in order to speak, he needed in fact to use me as a support, to be in complete harmony with my thoughts, as when we would look in the same direction and one of us would put into words a thought belonging to neither of us in particular. When we were face to face, this harmony was disrupted, and he lost the feeling that I shared in whatever he was thinking; we became separate, since he found he had to tell me of a desire he was feeling there and then, which I was not feeling and which I was unaware of in him. And when that happened, the indefinite support that came from me when we were side by side faded away, and his own thoughts, left to themselves, crumbled.

It was after about two years that this situation changed. What I find interesting in this development is the particular way dialogue arose between us. Speech directly addressed to somebody else in the form of requests grew out of a transformation of his play with the balls of plasticine, which became gradually linked with imaginary representations. It was as part of this play of imagination that his first requests were made: he became capable of asking me for something as long as this took place inside the imaginative space. In this connection, his activity with the balls of plasticine was crucial. After having recapitulated the toilet ritual with his father, where the balls of plasticine became first "poo-poo," then "toilets," he started to diversify the meaning of this accessory. One day they turned into "orange juices," which we had to put into glasses, and it was then that Louis asked me directly, "Do you want some orange juice?" Asking happened when the plasticine balls were transposed into metaphor, when the child, having been to the "toilets" in accordance with the father-based ritual, was able to construct a simulated situation focused on orange juice. This was the first of several changes, as Louis became capable of conceiving of links between different spaces, between entities and persons that were distinct and differentiated. After speaking of the father-and-"toilets" scenario in connection with his plasticine play, he established another link, between two different toilets: there were toilets near my consulting room, the men's and the women's being right opposite the table where we would pause to blow on the plastic beakers, and one day we happened to see a "lady" going in and closing the door. So we talked about the things she was doing (she's peeing, she's flushing, here she comes) and that we couldn't see. On that occasion, when we went into my room, Louis looked at the telephone and asked me to "telephone the lady." This was one of his very first explicit requests in a real setting. Since I knew the "lady" to be the secretary attached to a neighboring team, I dialed her extension, and he talked with her about the set of events that had taken place behind the closed door while he and I were sitting outside it. Not long afterward, he went back to playing hiding games, except that now he did it properly: he hid behind a cabinet while I pretended not to see him. It was after this series of linkages (the ritual with the father, the "lady" entering, then leaving the toilets, the encounter with her by telephone) that something in his speech was released. His whole play activity diversified. During our sessions, he started to construct very complex spaces, standing for home interiors known to him, his own room, his parents' bedroom, a room that belonged to a friend of theirs who would sometimes visit them. And now, each time he addressed me, he had no hesitation in asking me for whatever he wanted.

Form that point on, things were under way, language developed in all its dimensions, and Louis was able to speak of things that worried him (a man on a train "who was vomiting and peeing and with blood on him") or things about himself when he was out of my sight, such as a photo of him inside a frame, which he told me was usually kept "at home, in his house," as though he wanted to show me what he looked like when I was not with him. Clearly, this was all about his constructing his identity, his concern about my seeing permanence in him, in a way that enabled him to be at variance with me. He even reached the stage of calling me "you bastard." Next there came a development of the notion of distance and the possibility of separation, via a detailed account of the series of airplanes required to get to "his country," with many maneuvers carried out with different models of toy planes. Some time after that, just after New Year's Day, he brought me a little package tied with string, in which there was a New Year's wish; as he sat drawing, he sang to himself, "Draw me a child for life." Our games became more like standard childhood therapies. One day he took some toys out of his schoolbag (a transforming ball, a few cars) and told me Santa Claus was giving them to me but that a wicked witch was taking them away. I took my precautions against her, but he told me she had just killed me, to which I replied of course that under the ground I came back to life and found some of my pals, so he countered this by saying there was "another witch who killed me again." He hid behind the double curtains, as he had sometimes done before, came around behind me, with his face covered by the tulle, and grabbed me by the head as though to kill me. Some time later, he told me he had been thinking he might stay away from every second session but that now he intended to come every week. And he added, with a laugh, "I've got two Mr. Danon-Boileaus, one at home and one here." Soon after that, he also asked me the name of the child whose appointment time was just before his, who came, he believed, from a country close to his own. At the session after that, he had us take turns at drawing on a sheet of paper, which was then turned face down so that the one who had not done the drawing would have to guess what it was. By now we were in a processual mode, familiar to me from my field of childhood psychoanalysis. At the same time, the boy's language had similarly evolved in its forms: he was able to use "I" assertively, make up complicated negative structures, tell structured stories, and talk about events that were about to happen. Initially, when we looked out at the world, he had contrasted nearby things inside the consulting room with distant things seen outside the window. Then came our games with the plasticine, which had gradually taken on meaning. Using this fictional element, Louis had become able to organize separate spaces, that is to say, each of them rich in its own way with different, independent, and not necessarily contrasting stories. We now had the space we shared and his space "at home, in my house," but also a fictive space in which we could make up whatever happened. Through all this, he had attained the ability to assert himself and to display a measure of humor.

Counterpointing his moments of uncontroled outbursts, there were other more neutral activities, notably board games that we played. In these, he was often the winner, particularly when we played "Connect Four," in which he became extremely quick at detecting vertical, horizontal, and diagonal alignments, without further trouble with his eyesight.

What I Learned from Working with Louis

Like Ahlem, Lanny, and Simon (whose case I am coming to), Louis is one of the positive outcomes.

The boy's situation, seen as a problem of nosography, was not fundamentally different from Lanny's. The presence of autistic features was undeniable, but it would not have been proper to speak of autism. As with Lanny, this mitigated diagnosis was justified by the fact that it was possible to establish interaction with him at our very first session, when I folded over the piece of plastic fence in imitation of his action and he copied what I had done and then when I held out my hand and he gave me another piece without much prompting. A second promising sign was that I managed to make him smile during our exchanges. What was peculiar to him, though, was the importance of his faculty of eyesight within the general system of his cognitive process. It looked as though seeing for him was merely a way of noticing details and that he was unable to relate them to any broader field of vision. This much was evident, for instance, in the way he said "bread" of a dry sponge because that was what the small holes in it reminded him of. The same seemed true of the word "tortoise," which he applied to a plastic figure wearing a gored bonnet reminiscent of the wavy edge of the shell of some tortoises. In itself, the habit of young children of extending the name of an object to other, not dissimilar objects is unremarkable. Many toddlers will say "dog" of any animal with four legs, whether it is a dog, a wolf, a fox, or even at times a cow. But the thing I found intriguing with Louis was that for him it was an apparently irrelevant detail of the thing in question that made him make these conflations. In addition, his way of proceeding was not affected by any consideration of the basic object in its entirety. Here, too, one could legitimately wonder whether there was not some sort of dissociation at work, possibly related in some way to the simultagnosia observed in some neurological disorders of eyesight in adults, where details of shape cease to be perceived in relation to the broader context, leading to mistakes of interpretation. When we played hide-and-seek and he echoed my call of "Peekaboo" but did not come to find me, my impression there, too, is that what we are dealing with is a loss of linkage between elements of meaning, in this case between the sound sign ("Peekaboo") and the meaning given to the word by the game, which consequently is aborted. Apart from that, from the point of view of language, though Louis definitely presents a disorder in perception of language which is responsible for his way of stringing together incomprehensible utterances (his perception of phonemes is faulty and so is his reproduction of them), what was peculiar to him in his use of language was his way, in the early days of treatment, of talking essentially to himself. As I said, he had two registers of speech, two types of utterances that varied depending on what he was doing: either he whispered or he used his pedantic voice. Thus, his case shows once more the effect of a cognitive disorder on communication and language. And, as before, this disorder can be made sense of via the notion of "dissociation." However, though the "dissociation" is applicable to the three analogous impairments of Ahlem, Lanny, and Louis, it is important not to lose sight of the differences among them that it does not cover. The particular mode of dissociation visible in Louis affects him in the register of eyesight and in the ability to make different uses of language.

As a final passing remark, it can be said that Louis's earliest ventures into language (the fact that for quite a while he appeared to be more inclined to talk to himself than to me) also had an effect on theory: quite simply, it cast doubt on the received idea that in the development of language there is an initial phase in which what is used in dialogue resurfaces later in monologue and the stream of consciousness. In the case of Louis, what happened seemed to be the exact opposite.

9

Simon and the Magic Dictation

In the nineteenth century, it was commonly held that children's inner life and language were products of the richness of their exchanges within the family circle and that there could be nothing in a child's monologue with self that had not first emerged in dialogue with others. In an analogous way, it was taken for granted that oral language always came before writing and that only those children who were proficient in the spoken language could ever hope to become good readers. Though such common-sense principles may well be valid in the great majority of cases, there are notable exceptions that radically contradict some of our assumptions about the sequence of stages that have to be gone through by the notional baby we all have in mind when we try to understand and judge our everyday observation and treatment of children's speech disorders. In the story of Simon we see one such exception. Over the first four years of his treatment, I had to rethink some of my ideas about the necessary sequence of semiotic abilities crucial to the emergence of language. As will be seen, here was a little boy who was capable of spelling and reading before he could speak distinctly enough to be understood. Today, at almost eight years old, he speaks, though he has not fully developed expertise in verbal exchanges or a mode of speech that enables him to communicate easily with all interlocutors. If verbal exchange is to be possible with him, he needs to be treated with some considerateness by an interlocutor, as he is given to changes of subject and tone that can be very disturbing. Nevertheless, despite his agitation and the difficulty he has in abiding by rules within a group, he can be a part-time member of an ordinary class, and this enables him to make significant progress, though he does of course require teachers with a degree of tolerance.

The State of Simon's Speech

As I have said, dialogue with Simon is even now not quite natural, and I intend to outline here the ways in which this is apparent. First of all, there are constraints on the range of subjects that he can talk about. He can talk about anything in the immediate surroundings, but when he wants to speak about events from his past, he needs to be sure that I know about them and that I took part in them with him. Apart from that, he can talk about anything governed by a precise routine, ask questions, for example, about the near future (his own future or someone else's), as long as it can be seen as belonging to a repetitive routine. Curiously, though he always knows which day of the week it is and is familiar with the schedule of his activities set down for each weekday, he can neither grasp the meaning of "yesterday" and "tomorrow" nor talk about a particular past event that he experienced unaccompanied. The important thing here is that Simon is not yet able to indulge in idle chat or to speak for the mere enjoyment of it: in order to express what he wants or feels, there must be an element of necessity or even urgency in it. He mostly uses expressions that have a set formulaic character, such as "Don't want to," "Give me it," or "Leave me alone." But he can neither modulate what he means nor, of course, paraphrase his meaning. Essentially, Simon will not speak unless it is, in some way or other, "vital" that he do so.

In their content, his statements are obviously rather brief, though he does have, in addition to what is sometimes called "automatic" language (made up of set expressions, each of which corresponds to a particular inner sensation or a well-defined social situation), an "intentional" language. He makes sentences of at most two words, which may also contain some rudimentary syntax: *lèpati lavoitu* ("elle est partie, la voiture" = "car's gone"). This is about the most he can manage. Despite this, he can read: he can read out a text written in French; surprising though it may be, it is evident that he gleans some notion of what he produces in this way. It is this contrast of abilities that is the strange thing.

Diverse Readings of His Disorder

It is clear that, in Simon's language and communication, there are some very strange aspects. Any attempt to define the nature of these leads to contradictory results. For instance, there can be no doubt that he presents some "aphasiological" disorders akin to those found in children with ex-pressive disorder. This classification helps explain the fact that he has good "automatic" language (this includes exclamations and brief commands closely related to a given situation) and that his "intentional" language rarely runs to anything more than two signifying words. The efforts he makes when he tries to produce a statement of some length may also explain the hoarse-ness of his timbre and his labored diction. Also, as treatment advanced, he developed the ability to repeat quickly and easily long and complicated statements, which is rather rare in disorders of this type. If he recites some-thing he knows by heart, his speech changes in a way that blurs the con-tours of the words as he says them at high speed. No child with expressive disorder could be expected to have such ease of elocution even with some-thing learned by heart. When he is reading or reciting, it almost sounds as though his pathology changes category: there is a change of rhythm in his delivery, and his diction is so different that one could think one is listening to a child with receptive disorder. The important thing appears to be the relation between thought and spoken word: each time he tries to create meaning, his diction is that of the child with an expressive disorder; but when he recites something that he knows by heart or "reads a book," his speech sounds more like that associated with receptive disorder. At the start of treatment, he was more intelligible when he spelled out words from memory than when he tried to pronounce them.

In his cognitive profile, too, there are very marked disparities. In some ways, Simon has always been extremely alert: he watches over his mother; when they are on the *métro* and she goes to sleep, he recognizes the right station and wakes her up. Similarly, knowing she is supposed to take daily medication (she has a serious blood disorder), he makes a point of going and getting the boxes of pills from the medicine chest every morning at breakfast time and sets them out beside her place at the table. One sus-pects he has an inkling of their relation to life and death, to safety and danger: a few months into his treatment with me, in a bout of extraordi-nary violence, he swallowed a few tubes of pills and ended up in hospital having his stomach pumped out. So it would not be accurate to say that he lives in a world of his own or that he is incapable of attending to things outside himself. However, such attention as he is capable of mustering is strictly limited to certain areas; and there are even times when he seems to be completely incapable of it. Watching him play, I have on occasion seen him trying to force a large toy soldier into a tiny car, when he should have realized at a glance the difference in scale. This struck me as especially surprising because, when he was playing at fitting the Russian dolls inside one another, he seemed not to encounter that sort of difficulty and never once tried to insert one of the large ones into the body of a smaller one. In other cognitive areas, he shows analogous contradictions. For example, he knows how to roll a cloth ball, but he is unable to catch it if you throw it to him: he has no idea how to hold his hands, as though he finds it impossible to interpret the motions of the thrower or to foresee either the trajectory of the ball or the hand position required to catch it. This particular difficulty may suggest that he suffers from a disorder of intermodality, making him unable to convert visual information (the sight of the thrower's action) into postural information (he cannot tell which posture is required of his body if he is to catch the ball that he can see coming toward him). But there are other situations in which he can at times show aptitudes that are surprising in such a child. For example, he has no trouble converting tactile information into visual information: when he is feeling an object that he cannot see (a cube, a cone, a cylinder, a top, a rod), he is perfectly able to recognize the shape in question from an image and to single it out from the others.

The Psychological Climate

So much for Simon's difficulties. What needs to be stated now is especially the circumstances of his birth and the anxiety about his chances of survival and those of his mother. The fact was that, during her pregnancy, a routine examination showed she had a possibly life-threatening blood disorder that, if transmitted to her unborn child, might endanger his life, too. When she was told of this, she considered having an abortion. However, her husband was against this and threatened to leave her. Simon was two years old before the doctors could reassure her that the child had not contracted the disease. One can easily imagine the parents' extreme anxiety faced with a child whose life was so acutely threatened and the depression that must have colored the earliest exchanges with their son. Of itself, that could go a long way toward "explaining" many of the boy's difficulties, including at least his state of withdrawal, if not the actual absence of language. However, the mother was convinced that he was "autistic," and I had immense trouble in persuading her to abandon this conclusion, to which she had no doubt jumped after hearing the word bandied about by people in reference to her son.

Treatment: The Early Stages

After Simon's first session, which two of us therapists attended, our conclusions were very mixed: he had no language at all, and his nonverbal communication was very problematical; if things became ever so slightly tense, he would get into a state of agitation that ruled out any possibility of exchange, but his eye contact, the links we could establish with him during settled moments, and the understanding attitude of the school he attended made us suspect that, though it would undoubtedly be difficult for him to learn to relate to others, it might not be impossible.

At that first session, after Simon had played by himself for a while, he started to take an interest in us: my (female) colleague had set out a row of fences in front of him, and he ran a toy car around them. A little later, I showed him how you could make the car move by blowing it along, and this he found very amusing. When the car reached the edge of the table, I told him to run it back to me, and he did so; when it was my turn to roll it back to him, I added a slight complication to the game by counting to three so that he could be ready for my action. All this had gone very well, and these simple exchanges had convinced us that we could get the boy to respond to treatment. Despite his difficulties, he had the ability to engage in a game with an unfamiliar adult, which revealed something of his link to the world of others and suggested that further treatment could well lead to a favorable outcome. As far as speech was concerned, of course, he had said not a word, merely humming bits of songs to himself during his solitary play. Against that, though, there was the fact that when I started to whistle along with him, he was both surprised and pleased.

Two weeks later, at the second session, our feeling that he was going to be able to engage in full exchange was confirmed. (We made up a game in which he first drew circles, and then, at a sign from him, I put a dot inside them.) He even remembered the previous session: before running the car toward me, he spontaneously started to count. We also heard him speak rather than sing, as he accompanied his own actions with a word of encouragement, *Bravo* (= "Good!"), that I had often said to him the previous time. And when he did sing, though the words were deformed, one could still recognize the rhythm and the tune. Overall, the child seemed to enjoy playing in our presence—I put it like that, rather than say "playing with us," because I had the impression that we still represented a kind of atmosphere for him and not quite two people endowed with clear contours.

The format of treatment was quickly organized. His mother told us she could be part of it, but for only one session a week. Because she had problems in her ways of relating unaided to the child, we decided they should come to the consultations together, in the hope that this might afford her the enjoyment of an exchange with him untroubled by any of the educative concern—the urge to make the child speak—that seemed to inspire everything she said or did when with him.

Progress in Interaction

So the four of us met once a week. In one way, the sequence was standard in that Simon was interested in hiding games (he readily said "Peekaboo" on coming out of his hiding place); then he took to pointing, indicating, for example, the ascending line of the Russian dolls, going from the smallest to the tallest; when I drew a man's head, naming in turn the mouth, the eyes, and the other features, he touched his head when I said "hair." This evidence suggested that he was going through a speeded-up version of the usual development of a young child between the ages of eight months and a little over eighteen months. While he was making this progress, he was also showing unexpected abilities that were in marked contrast to this suggestion of catching up. For example, he would spend much time in counting. He could count up to thirty and got angry if I gave the impression I was going to count with him. He saw my counting with him as an attempt to help him, as an infringement of his independence; he resisted this as a reminder of the deficiencies that marked him as a child with difficulties.

Fragmentary as this evidence was, behind it there was visibly a mind at work, though it expressed itself in ways that were not always well formulated. For example, on a day when I was a little late in arriving, not seeing me in the waiting room, he went out to the elevators and pressed as hard as he could on the buttons, as though this would make me appear by magic. He was capable, too, of surprising acts of considerateness: his mother told us that, the previous evening, when she got home very tired from work, he had taken her to her bed, tucked her in, and said, "Go bye-bye." In a sudden realization of her child's particular sensitivity, she said, "It was as though he was trying to console me." That a child who had so much trouble "communicating," even through sign language, should give such an appropriate response to an adult's emotional state is nothing short of remarkable. In such a circumstance, what does "communicating" actually mean? What difference would there be between Simon's miming, with his "Go bye-bye," and what a teenager might say to his mother with a kiss: "Go and lie down; you need a rest"? It makes complete sense to see Simon's way of acting toward his mother as the expression of an intention in every way comparable to that. It is not true, however, to say that all he was doing was putting the same idea into mime. Even if we leave aside his purely linguistic difficulties, how can we make sense of the disparity between his ability to empathize and his frequent lack of elementary communication by movement and gestures? Part of the answer lies, no doubt, in the fact that what he was signifying was the expression of what he felt, rather than an intended input to a reasoned exchange within a stable and controlled relationship with another person. His various actions of this sort say something about his reactions, his wishes, and his affective state. They were neither signs meant as part of an exchange nor a mode of stabilized communication. Basically, the child was trying not to make himself understood but to express himself. Then there were other moments when his play became even more complicated through his possession of special aptitudes.

The Magic Dictation

The following is an account of an event that took place shortly before the summer interrupted our meetings and that seems to me to be related to the special aptitudes I speak of. His mother told us one day that he could read and spell out words, that he played with his big brother's "magic dictation" and was pretty good at it. Magic Dictation, a computerized educational game for children going into first grade, is a pocket PC that shows a picture of an object on a little screen while a synthesized voice says the name of it. When the child presses the letters on the keyboard to spell the word, they appear one by one under the picture. If the spelling is correct, the computer says approvingly, "That's right"; if it is not correct, it orders the child to do it again. This process continues until either the spelling is right or the child has had enough and presses the button that gives the right answer.

When the boy's mother told us of Simon's magic dictation exploits, we were rather disturbed and skeptical, and we wanted to see the game so as to judge for ourselves. She brought it to the next session, but each time it asked the child to put in a letter, all he did was press "h," and we concluded that she had been indulging in wishful thinking. Nevertheless, a week later, Simon was back with the game, and this time he could spell everything: every time the computer showed a picture and spoke the word, he pressed the right letters. Or, if he did not know the spelling, he pressed the button for the right answer, then touched each of the letters on the keyboard as the computer spoke them. It had taken him a week to learn this whole process. When we expressed our astonishment to his mother, she explained that he had typed in only "h" the last time because his magic dictation was a new one, he having broken the previous one in a tantrum. It was time to continue with the session, but it proved impossible to do anything other than watch him play with his computer. When his mother tried to take it away, he threw a tantrum of such violence that we had to give in and let him sit under the table, where he went on calling out words nonstop and spelling them. Toward the end of the session, as he had settled down a little, I started to write up on the board the words displayed by the computer (*douze, mille, cent, nez* = twelve, thousand, hundred, nose). This I did exactly as the computer had done it: I spoke each word, then I spelled it out letter by letter, and when I had finished I said "Good!" in the same tone as that used by the child. Gradually, I brought in other words related to his family, his name, the names of his father, his mother, and a little girl who lived near him. This got him interested, so he came out from under the table and wanted to have a turn at writing on the board. At first I guided his hand; then I encouraged him to write unaided, and when he managed to do so, he was glad to see that what he had written was readable. His mother was the one to echo the computer's congratulations: "Good, Simon!"

We found this disparity between the child's learning abilities by computer and his retarded language quite intriguing, though there is no shortage of hypotheses that might explain it. It might be, for instance, that the shape of the letters had a helping effect on pronunciation: his ability to spell, to clearly enunciate the name of each letter, despite his inability to pronounce whole words, might come from the fact that each letter pronounced separately corresponded to an easily identifiable written form and that this form stabilized his pronunciation, whereas because he could not yet read whole words, he could draw no benefit from silent recognition of them. His memory for the written word was not good enough. So it would appear that he could not correctly pronounce a signifier unless his recognition of the phonemes could be supported by a single item of knowledge of which he had a full grasp. This item might be the image of a letter, a tune, or a fixed situation (such as those in which he could say "Good" or "Hello"). What he could not manage to do was give utterance to an idea or a notion unassociated with an image or an action of small scope, presumably because that would have required recognition of a signifier from sound accompanied by nothing else, the sort of recognition that could happen unaided and be available for the evocation of an idea. It was not yet possible for him to let ideas be expressed as words. In order to do that, he would have needed to be able to find words unsupported by anything, so that there could be a flexible correspondence between thinking and putting things variously into words. It is only in that type of situation that a word can be the translation into voice of an idea that remains latently variable and expressible in different ways. For the time being, Simon could pronounce a sound only if it was associated with an action, an image, or a set situation. It was this association that enabled him to speak the word.

It quickly became apparent that the game centered on the little computer would lead nowhere unless we could contrive to turn it into a medium of exchange. The thing to do was to find a way of adapting the words spoken by the machine to some association with feelings or moving pictures. This was apparent to the boy's mother too, for she, like us, was bothered by this uncanny ability of Simon's in the use of language. It struck her as surprising, for example, that he should be able to remember without difficulty television commercials, despite having such trouble in communicating, as though he paid attention only to words spoken by machines but not to anything that interested human beings might want to tell him. That his mother was now able to share with others her feeling about the strangeness of her son's mind seemed to us a good sign; we made no secret of the fact that we too were rather perplexed by his abilities. They could not be explained by the fact that he spent too long sitting by himself in front of the television or by the suggestion that he felt less threatened by machines than by people (even though this might be true). However, one peculiarity of television commercials should not be overlooked: by simplifying and stylizing reality, they are much easier to take in. They isolate a particle of reality; they frame it and focus on it. They have only two dimensions, not three. They proceed via changes that are quick and coherent (affecting image and sound simultaneously). And they deal in situations to which the viewer is not required to respond. The viewer sits facing images, out of contact with any real human being. Not to mention, of course, the fact that they go on reappearing, identical every time.

With the approach of summer, at the session after the one with the magic dictation, we talked about the coming interruption in treatment. Simon's mother was saying she wanted him to go and spend a few days in the country so that she could have a rest but that she was unsure whether he could cope with this, and while she was speaking about it, the child made up a new game: he kept coming into the room, then going out again. At each disappearance, he went on a brief exploration of our premises, then came back. My colleague commented on this as symbolic practicing for the coming separation, but also as a change in the child's attitude, showing that he was now able to leave us and rejoin us. The mother also remarked that he was now making efforts to speak.

At the final session for the school year, we took up our spelling games at the board, based as before on the model of the magic dictation. By now, Simon was repeating much more readily the words I spoke and spelled for him, such as *voiture* (= "car"), which he repeated after me and spelled out, so that I could write up the letters at his dictation. I had become him; he had become not only me but the computer, as well. Then he spoke, quite clearly, the word *soleil* (= "sun"), and I drew a sun. He spelled out the letters, and I wrote them out as he dictated them. My colleague announced that this was the end of the session, saying, "It's over." I wrote up the word *fin* (= "the end") and drew a circle around it. Then, as I said "Au revoir," I wrote that up, too, and as he shook my hand at the door, Simon said, "Au revoir." We were left with the feeling that, what with the computer, the games, and our role in it, some broader contact had been made on the matter of separations.

A Change and the Reasons for It

The changes that had come about were the outcome of my own substantial but limited intervention in Simon's ritual of the magic dictation. Two essential things, it seems to me, happened when I contrived to get into his game.

The first was that I managed to weave together two hitherto separate and closed rituals, the one focused on his spelling of the words dictated by the computer and the one related to the rather automatic "Au revoir" that he said as we shook hands at the end of each session. In fact, as the episode of the words *Au revoir* written up on the board had happened right at the end of the session and immediately before our separation for the summer, the two words, by being both spoken and written, had suddenly acquired an affective charge that gave them back their full content of meaning (= "till we see each other again"). This, I think, was a decisive shift: the written word and the spoken word had taken on their proper meaning within a moment of genuine sharing.

The other thing, equally essential in my view, had happened earlier, when Simon agreed to dictate the words to me so that I could spell them out for him and write them up, in imitation of the computer ritual. By dictating the words, he was in effect manipulating and controlling my thinking and its results (my spelling out loud and my written transcription of it) as he had been doing with the computer. By acting the part of the computer, I gave him the feeling that he could control my thinking; this simulation of manipulation and mastery helped him (at any rate, this is the sense I see in it) to alter his way of engaging with my mind.

In everyday living, the thinking of each individual is emblematic of that person's autonomy and otherness. Thinking for oneself is what makes it possible for someone else to leave you at a moment's notice, lose interest in you, take an interest in somebody other than you, and dump you. Any hint of thought in another person confirms the fact that he or she may disappear on the spur of a momentary whim. This is why it is hard to relate to another mind except as a source of displeasure, why others' thinking is essentially dangerous, and why one may hate it. Hating others' thinking is the basic obstacle to using any subject's thought for play. It takes a long apprenticeship to learn that one has no control over others' thinking and that, though the potential absence of the other is inevitable, this does not rule out taking pleasure in relating to others. Of course, one may never reach that stage; one may merely hate the thinking of the other or behave as though it does not exist. Neither of these makes for ease of communication or for a partiality for language. In fact, in order to foster the emergence of language in a child with a disorder, it is necessary to let him engage differently with the minds of others. Such children must be given the opportunity of manipulating other people's thinking. And, in my view, that was what happened when Simon dictated words and I wrote them out for him just like a computer. In that way, he was manipulating and controlling my thinking and its results (my speech and my action) as he had done with the computer when I had been imitating it. Another thing that was crucial in this game was the fact that I did not touch him. It was because we did not touch each other that the child exercised control over my mind and not just over my body.

After the Separation

By the start of the new school year, major changes had taken place. Simon made up new games: when all four of us went into the consulting room, he pushed me out again and shut the door on me, excluding me as he presumably felt he had been excluded during the summer. I turned this into a game, by knocking on the door so that he could open it and allow me in. During the vacation he had been placed with a foster family and went home with his mother on the weekends, an arrangement that had worked out very well. She was well aware of how her son had changed: "He calls me *maman* now. He has also started saying proper sentences to ask me for a piece of bread, corn flakes, or a drink of milk, and when I can't understand him, he keeps trying, he repeats what he's just said." As a result of a separation that had turned out well, the child now had the ability to express and communicate his desires and had become a symbolic subject for the mother. Now that she felt recognized as a mother by a child who called her *maman*, she found she could also consider him as a human being with a wish to communicate. What was also noticeable was that, during our session, the boy was much more attentive to what was being said in his presence; more than once he took up and elaborated on things his mother was telling us. When she told us how he spoke when he wanted something to eat, he took a plate and a fork from a tea set and pretended to eat with them; when she told us he could count to five hundred, he started counting to show us what he could do. A little later, as though to mark this occasion of our reunion, he took up again all the games we had played before the vacation. He asked me to write; if I started drawing instead of writing, he got angry. If I wrote *papa, maman, Simon*, he showed his approval, then went and got the Russian dolls and fitted them together. As he played, he uttered nonstop cheerful lallations, like those of a younger child, except that they were full of clearly sounded consonants. Here, too, I noticed a change: his way of relating to the dolls was no longer just to assemble them like so many shapes; and when he handled the smallest one, he called it "baby." Then, as before, he asked me to draw a face, and repeated after me the word for each feature as it was drawn in: the nose, the mouth, the eyes, the ears, and, last, the hair, which I drew as a squiggly garland, thus affording him much amusement. It must have been the shape of it that made him laugh, for when my colleague depicted the smoke rising from a normal chimney with a similar squiggle, she got the same result from him. Later, when she drew smoke coming from another chimney, he said, "Hair." Some of his cognitive difficulties persisted, as seen, for example, in his inability to find a particular car in the toybox, though it was visible, albeit jumbled up among all the other toys. It looked as though the tangling together of different shapes blurred the image in a way that made the outline of the car unrecognizable to him.

In addition to all this, the magic dictation was still very much with us, as was the spelling of the names of objects; so, by way of some relief, I suggested that we try a hand with the "Memory" cards, the image-pairing game that we had played once or twice before the separation, at which Simon had been pretty good, though he never seemed interested by the representational quality of the pictures. He would look for a picture, find the one that matched, and put them together, but he never reacted to the images, either by word or by action. Now, though, he studied a picture of an ice cream cone in which a drop of ice cream was overflowing the top of the cone: he fingered the drop, licked his fingertip, and pretended to eat the drop of ice cream, while hiding it on the picture. This action made us suddenly realize that his whole relation to graphic signs had been transformed: previously, when he turned over a "Memory" card, he had been incapable of doing anything other than putting two similar pictures together; now he could play with a picture, run his finger over it, convey the finger to his mouth. To my mind, the essential thing here was a sequence of stages: my being the computer had been a crucial development, necessary for the emergence in the child of an ability to use images as representations and not just a set of lines. It was as though there had been a change in his relation to signs, dating from his discovery of his ability to transform me into a computer, to use my representation, to make me speak, move my wrist, and exercise a kind of remote control over my thinking, as though he and I were jointly in charge of it all.

Through this experience of thought control, Simon was enabled to engage with my mind, my speech, and my action in ways that made them no longer just signs of my unbearable otherness. Having seen into my ability to represent, he was then able to construe a graphic image as something more than a mere set of fixed lines, as something that I, too, might be able to see as the sign of an inner representation. An image can, in fact, become a sign once it can give rise to a common representation in two people looking at it simultaneously. They can then exchange, via word and gesture, views on this representation, though its physical presence amounts only to the graphic signs. In other words, for an image to be representative, each of the two people looking at it must think that the other is thinking and that the other's thinking, though different from one's own, can be relied upon. This means that the other's thinking must have stopped being emblematic of an unbearable otherness. After he had used my thinking, Simon was able to have the idea that an image stands for a representation in the mind of another human being. The "Memory" card became the sign of a representation that was sharable with me, which was what enabled him to finger the picture of ice cream with a smile of amusement and relish. The image was not just an assemblage of lines but stood for something else; the thing that gave it this new nature, the thing that guaranteed this make-believe dimension of it, was the fact that for me, too, it stood for something other than a mere picture, as well as the fact that the child, from his experience of controlling my thinking, had acquired an intuitive certainty of what I thought.

Simon's General Evolution and the Questions It Raises in Hindsight

Nosographically speaking, Simon belongs (as do Lanny, Louis, and Rachid, a boy of whose treatment I spoke in *The Silent Child*, chapter 4) to the category of childhood psychosis. However, unlike the outcome with the three others, Simon's later evolution, though remarkable in many ways, did not lead to a return to normal life and the possibility of taking up ordinary schooling and eventually being assimilated without particular precautions into society. My present feeling is that Simon will be able to find a place in society all right but that it will always need to be a sheltered place. With him, leaving aside the developments that came out of the magic dictation, there were many surprises and discoveries. One question, though, remains unanswered in my mind: even with the benefit of hindsight, rereading the notes I made at the outset, was his evolution foreseeable? Should I have suspected that it would be different from Lanny's, Louis's, and Rachid's? Rewriting history is always tempting, once one knows how things did turn out. Honesty constrains me to admit my ignorance: to this day, quite frankly, when I collate my notes from the earliest sessions with all four of these children, I can see nothing that might make it possible to say, "This is a clue that should have made me suspect that the first three would make remarkable progress; and that is a very different clue that should have alerted me to the worrying likelihood that with Simon things were going to be much harder." When nothing else is noteworthy about a child, there is always the rather facile expedient of looking for a clue in the family circumstances. Simon's family was not as close-knit as those of the other three boys, and his father was less in evidence. One important factor that was a source of serious anxiety for the boy was his mother's health. Though the effects of this on his general evolution could not be ascertained, it was conceivable, for example, that he might have formed the notion that, if he could stop growing up, this would oblige his mother to go on living so as to continue being the essential intermediary between himself and the rest of the world. From this point of view, if he ever did fully accept his own growing up and allowed himself to become psychically independent, he would be letting his mother die. There is presumably some truth in this way of defining his plight, but it is rather too rough-hewn and could justify many different conclusions. Also, paradoxically, the problems he continues to have to this day are more closely related to his use of language than to his ways of communicating. His language continues to be essentially automatic speech composed of set expressions. One can get the impression that his only intentional speech happens through written words, as used to be the case when he was reading a book or deciphering his magic dictation on a screen. He can actually engage in intentional speech, though this works only with something that is devoid of affect, such as giving the answer to a classroom question. If there is the slightest emotion entailed in what is to be said, he finds it impossible to program any intended utterance before speaking it. Even though he has made great progress in his spontaneous language, which has become broader and more diverse, any statements he makes continue to be disjointed, as though his utterances are the result of faulty associations between "lumps of speech" that belong to diverse registers and different situations. My own impression, possibly inaccurate, is that it is the mechanical component of his language that prevents him from using speech to temper his emotions and think calmly. What he does use it for is to give violent expression to pleasure, displeasure, or discontent, to formulate a request, or to voice an anxiety, but he is incapable of modulation. His use of language serves in no way to filter, socialize, or develop his world of innermost sensation.

So, what could possibly have led me to expect difficulties of this kind? In our very first sessions, there was manifestly next to nothing, since he said hardly anything and whatever he did say was in the register of automatic speech. Perhaps the magic dictation episode should have made me realize that the outlook was not as optimistic as I was inclined to think. The fact that, though the child was able to spell out words, he was unable to speak them ought to have made me foresee a considerable impairment in his ability to produce intentional speech.

In retrospect, all I can do is acknowledge the fact that Simon has made great progress, both in language and in his ability to engage in exchange, while acknowledging also my own uncertainties about what it might have been in his evolution that forever prevented him from enjoying normal schooling. Nowadays he is in early adolescence, and I still see him regularly once a week. He continues to make progress in his schooling, a process that will continue for some time. When we play at "Connect Four," he is often the winner.

10

Charles, or Paradoxical Communication

All the consultants agreed about Charles: by the age of six, he was still not speaking, and there was a definite autistic element in his disorder. With him, play was out of the question. However, as will be seen, his ability with signs was particularly rich and complex, and he was well able to show what he wanted. This paradoxical dimension was what made working with him as exciting as it was difficult. To tell the truth, of all the children described in this book, Charles was the one whose symptoms most closely corresponded to a definite diagnostic category: his disorder was autism without language. However, like other children with this disorder, he could still make himself understood via writing. This was what I found most interesting, as it meant he must be credited with a functioning mind. This ruled out naive and simplistic notions, such as that autistic children do not have "any representations or any representation of another person's mind." As can often happen, clinical practice leads to a more complex way of seeing things. Needless to say, my acceptance that there was a mind at work in this child did not mean that I assumed everything would be plain sailing from then on. The first thing that came to my own mind was a question: since he does have a mind that works, why does he not make more use of it to establish a bond with others?

Here, first, is an event that shows how extremely complex the situation was. During an earlier session, the boy had seen a toy car in a different consulting room and wanted to play with it again this time. The door was closed, and he worked at the knob to no avail. As a last resort, he looked at me and made the action of sawing through the door, imitating the regular movement of the sawyer's arm. I being slow to respond, he ran back into our own room, took a picture book, and opened it at the page that showed a small handsaw. He made the movement of gripping it by the handle and stared at me. How could one best characterize the thinking that had led him to this sequence of acts? What representation did he have of me? It was clear that he could see how futile his efforts were and that, for all his desire that the door should open, it had remained shut. He had also grasped the fact that his pretense of sawing through the door had not managed to make any inroads on it. He had further realized that, by having recourse to different figurations of a saw, he could make me understand that he wanted to be rid of the obstacle preventing him from getting at the car. From this perspective, it must be accepted that, despite his language handicap, he knew how to use symbolization. It is quite remarkable, for example, that he did not resort to throwing tantrums, burst into tears, or kick at the door. Here was a child who was capable of symbolizing through actions. Not only that; his use of symbolization made the distinction between the symbol and what is symbolized. He did not take scissors, for instance, to cut out the picture of the saw and try to hold it by the handle. Nor was he the type of child who walks around behind a picture to look for the other side of the thing depicted. Nevertheless, in his way of using the picture of the saw, it was not completely a sign. Though for him the picture was distinct from the referent constituted by the saw, it did not make the standard link between signifier and signified. To him, what the picture meant was "I demand that you go and get a saw and use it to destroy the door that prevents me from playing with the toy car on the other side of it." The sign was a sort of imperative statement, not a declarative one. This was a constant mark of Charles's way of thinking: he had significant difficulty in engaging with any representation as such, as an object conducive to play, for instance. For him, symbolization, even complex symbolization, was of interest only insofar as it enabled him to achieve real gratification. No act with regard to it had meaning other than as possibly promoting actual access to the referent. A drawing of a saw led to no play: it was out of the question to pretend to break it, repair it, buy it, or sell it. Make-believe for the sake of make-believe was inconceivable. If he simulated anything, it was only as a way of showing me what he wanted to see really happen. The fictionality of such an act was acknowledged as such, of course, but was seen only as a device that might lead directly or indirectly to the fulfillment of a desire. The symbol was a simple instrument, like a number. Normally, the quality of the signs used by a child to communicate or share a representation gives one an appreciation of the way he came to make the representation; the relationship he can establish between his desires, reality, and someone else's mind is pretty apparent. With Charles, however, none of this was readily apparent. On the one hand, he never once took a drawing of a thing for the thing itself. So one can say that he was not hallucinating, that he did not think the sign and the object were one. He made no "symbolic equation," as Hanna Segal puts it, between the symbol and what it symbolized (Segal 1957). Against that, though, his way of appealing to me for a "real saw" as a way of getting rid of the door showed that he had not developed his fantasy of immediate destruction of the obstacle into something else. To make better sense of the situation he was in, we must draw upon certain themes from childhood psychoanalysis, in particular Melanie Klein's idea of the "depressive position." Roughly speaking, this states that, in normal cases, any subject who desires starts to fantasize, which constitutes both a necessity and a setback. If there is no fantasizing, there can be no project; but if the fantasizing remains undeveloped, there can be no real fulfillment. Before the work of thinking can begin, the subject must recognize the partially illusory nature of the fantasy, but without completely abandoning it. This complex process can function only through the "depressive position," which enables the suspension of the urge to immediate gratification and brings the project into a state that is compatible with the constraints of reality. Reason becomes ruse. As for Charles, on the one hand, as I have said, though he was not completely under the illusion of being all-powerful and did not deal with the drawing as though dealing with a real saw, on the other hand his fantasy was not properly developed; it remained in its crude and socially unacceptable state. This is what shows he had not yet achieved the full "depressive position." The reasons for this, which were presumably numerous, remained to be discovered. Perhaps play did not provide him with sufficient pleasure or support. Perhaps he was far too indifferent to whatever others had to offer. Perhaps he was simply full of hatred toward any thinking that was independent, autonomous, and different from his own. There are children with whom one can have a mode of signifying play and exchange that does not quite amount to the real thing. Their grasp of the relation between symbol and what is symbolized is sound; they make no equation between them. And, yet, their intolerance of others is such that anything that might turn into play is immediately frozen into a sequence of interminably repeated acts.

What Charles Could Do

So Charles's thinking was well developed and he had a measure of aptitude for communication. To gauge that aptitude (including its limits and its particularities) was, of course, the first aim of therapeutic intervention. The complexity of this task can be appreciated from an account of some of the major events that marked his course of treatment. To this day, the child still does not speak and seldom communicates; when he does communicate, it is only through mime and sign language. Mostly, though, he avoids eye contact and immerses himself in activities that no one else is allowed to participate in. So, when he comes into the consulting room, he goes on doing whatever he was doing in the waiting room, drawing, building something out of Legos, doing a jigsaw puzzle. My presence disturbs him, but he continues to play as I watch. What he likes to do is match things with one another or build replicas and counterparts of things. One day, having made a Lego model of the rooster pictured on the box, he went to get paper and a marker so as to draw a copy of the animal already made out of the little bricks: the thing represented must be accompanied by a picture of itself, in an effort to reduce space. Things must also be accompanied by words: I have seen him take a beaker of coffee out of his father's hands so as to place it carefully at the very spot where he had just written "coffee" on a piece of paper. To his mind, a written word does not stand for the thing: it must be inseparable from it. There was a time when he was fascinated by dictionaries of all sorts: most of the session would be spent with him looking up words, which he would then copy out, even juxtaposing them with the equivalent word in English. Throughout this play with counterparts, the whole process would take place in my presence without my being able to take any part in it. However, on occasion, he did include me: he once happened to open a book at a picture of a cow, whereupon he waited for me to speak the word; then he set about finding a toy cow among our playthings and finally wrote the word on the board.

Agitation Produced by Exchange

Now and again, moments of genuine exchange could happen, though they were few and far between, unfortunately. The fact that they always put the child into a state of agitation may explain why he never managed to develop them or make them the basis of more regular communication. So they were unforeseeable; the way they suddenly happened was incomprehensible; and the reasons why he stopped clinging to his self-sufficient solitude were inscrutable. Nor could one understand why such moments commonly led to nothing. There was, for example, a day when he took a marker and did a drawing on the board: it was a rectangle divided vertically into two compartments, in each of which there were two characters, with cords slanting downward. Supposing it was a sort of cable, I drew in a mountain. But the rectangle was then rounded and opened out into a kind of parachute, so I drew an airplane and a second parachute. Charles was so delighted at being understood that he jumped backward, but he was in such a state of agitation that he banged against the wall, burst into tears, and tried to leave. Then he caught sight of his reflection in the chrome finger plate on the door, which calmed him down a little and helped him to withdraw from the exchange, which he did by coiling up in a fetal position on the floor. I started drawing a doleful face, with tears under the eyes and the mouth turned down; then I put a lump on top of the head and wrote *Charles* underneath. He got up and came over to the board, where he erased first the lump, then the rest of the face. This all but put an end to our exchange, presumably because I had too clearly identified the character in tears and made him want to rub it out. Nevertheless, the exchange did not completely peter out: it took a new turn when I wrote under the different parts of our drawing what they represented (e.g., cloud, tree, mountain). Charles started drawing a row of crosses, which looked rather like a barrier, so I drew lines linking them together, but this was not to his liking. He drew another cross, slightly apart from the ones already drawn, and wrote *No*. I saw the meaning of his procedure: his crosses were signs like those one finds on preprinted forms; he was assessing my interpretations of his drawing by distributing zeros and crosses over the board. Beside the crosses, I wrote *No*; beside the zeros, I wrote *Yes*. The exchange proceeded in a fairly cheerful atmosphere. He then drew an airplane similar to mine, with windows and passengers. Under the ones near the front, I wrote *pilot* and *copilot*; under some of the others I wrote *Laurent*, *Charles*, *maman*, and *papa*. We were communicating.

A Birthday, with Plasticine

A sharing of affect was beginning to emerge, showing itself not only in these drawing games. For example, one evening when I went to find him in the waiting room, he was reluctant to come to the consulting room and hung back. When I insisted, he became very angry, took a Lego airplane that he had built, and dashed it to the floor. I picked up the scatter of pieces and put them into the pocket of my shirt. Eventually, not without a show of temper, he settled down a bit and came with me. When we got into the room, he went to the board and spontaneously wrote *stop*, as though he was asking me to restrain his aggressive impulses. So I drew the traffic sign meaning "danger," with a car, a street crossing, and a house. He then drew an airplane, to which I added a sun and then the word *airplane*, which I put in a corner of the board because he prevented me from writing it anywhere near him. Next, he came over to take the key of the cupboard out of my shirt pocket; when I pretended to be unhappy about this, he wrote the word *key*. As he went over to the toy cupboard, I found I was whistling "Happy Birthday to You"; quite spontaneously, he took out the plasticine, which he made into a cake and candles. Having first switched off the light, to set the scene properly, he even blew on the candles; then, once he had blown them out, he switched the light on again. Coming back to the board, he wrote up *Fête* (= "party" or "birthday"). Much moved by all this, I took him in my arms and congratulated him, something that upset him dreadfully. He struggled free of my arms and fell screaming and yelling to the floor. As before, I drew a grumpy face, with tears and a lump on the head. He erased first the lump, then the tears, and changed the mouth to make it smile, not saying anything. Then he drew a cloud and some rain; as he was putting in the strokes for the rain, I made up a little song to the rhythm of them. I wrote *nuage* ("cloud") beside the cloud and *il pleut* ("it's raining") beside the falling rain. A further elaboration was added to the scenario when he brought over some more plasticine: I modeled it into a knife and fork, which he used in a pretense of slicing up the cake. More than once during this, he started humming "Happy Birthday to You." This was a real sharing of play and feelings.

Compassion

When a child like Charles manifests such a great disorder in communication and resorts so often to withdrawal, one might expect that he would never reach the stage of displaying any affect, and certainly that he would never take notice of anyone else's. But that was not always the case with him. Although his affect was often masked by a rapid onset of agitation, there were occasions when this did not prevent him from being sensitive to my state of feeling. For instance, one day, wearied by his agitation and in some dismay at my own inability to establish contact with him, I sat down on the couch, with a sigh that was deeper than it should have been. He came over to me quietly, gave me a questioning look, lifted up my glasses, and with his fingers made the trickling of imaginary tears down my cheeks. He gave me a forced smile, as though wishing away my discontent and inviting me to smile back at him. So he had sensed my dejection, wanted to know my feelings, and inquired about them using a sign, while his eyes questioned me on the meaning of the emotion he thought he could detect in me. So communication through affect was present.

What Charles May Think about Others' Thinking

Charles was therefore capable of playing with and feeling for somebody else. What remained unclear, however, was how he related to somebody else's thinking. He was certainly capable of glancing toward the lock on the door while drawing a key and of giving me a sidelong look, as though trying to find support in my mind for the connections he made between sign and object. But, at the same time, he never pointed at anything, or, rather, never spontaneously. What difference was there between a child who points and a child like Charles who relies on furtive glances? What significance should be given to such a peculiar way of indicating? Was his abnormality affecting the nature of the act of signifying or only the form it took? One hypothesis might be, for instance, that Charles did not point because he could not manage to do two things at once, which is an essential skill if one wants to point, since pointing means paying attention to what interests you while attending to the mind of somebody else. It entails using one's finger to draw attention to something interesting and showing that one also engages with what someone else is thinking, that one cares about what another person is interested in, and that one is appealing to that other person. Pointing must thus link the displaying of one's own interest for someone else with an attempt to stimulate the latter's interest. And perhaps it was this dual movement that the child was incapable of. This first properly occurred to me when we were using a picture book. The game was that, as we turned the pages, Charles had me name the pictures. He was sitting beside me, a position in which it was plain to him that we were both looking in the same direction. There was thus no need for him to attract my interest. All he had to do was focus it on what he wanted me to look at so that we could be agreed on the object of our joint attention. To do this, he took my finger and pointed with it, as though my hand was an essential accessory to his drawing something to my attention. As a way of pointing, this is peculiar; it reminded me of another child who, when he wanted me to open the door for him, would take my hand and put it on the doorknob. Even so, Charles was not expecting me to manipulate the picture like a tool. As can be seen, it can be difficult to define a child's nonverbal communication. It might be thought that in his mind he was just identifying one thing with another, as in his juxtapositions of object with drawing or drawing with written word, as though trying to conflate everything into a single agglomerate. Yet, against that, he was sensitive to others' feelings; he could actually convey his anxiety about my sadness and ask me whether I was crying. And, occasionally, new scenarios would develop, though when communication of good quality did take place, it was still extremely difficult to grasp what determined the advent of it. This would often happen after a moment of marked conflict with me: once the atmosphere relaxed, he could make associations and start to play.

Curiously enough, Charles also had a sense of time. He could link events with dates. On one occasion, his father told me how, Charles having been promised that, on the Sunday of the week following, he could go and eat at McDonald's, the boy had taken a McDonald's advertising leaflet across to the calendar hanging on the kitchen wall and put it on the proper date. The relation between the event "going to McDonald's" and the right date was obvious. As our sessions progressed, it became clear that, despite moments of genuine exchange, the construction of a shared and continuing experience with him was no easy thing. Most of the time, he was immersed in a project, and if I attempted to divert him from it, he became agitated and lost the thread of his thoughts. It occurred to me, during discussions with colleagues, that Charles was afraid of forgetting the immediate past but that it came back to him spontaneously after a period of latency and discontinuity. This could explain why he often ignored suggestions of mine, only to take them up some time later, after I had abandoned them. It was the fear of forgetting the immediate past that compelled him into his repetitions. But it had an effect on me, too, giving me the feeling of having lost touch with our shared experience. I also noticed that with him, unlike what would happen with other children, I seldom found occasion to bring back into play objects that were reminders of our shared past, as though the child's difficulty in retaining his immediate past had inhibited my own ability to retrieve and use our common experiences. It is a simple fact that a child's disorders can hinder the mental processes of the therapist.

Part IV

Theoretical Foundations

11

Language and Symbolization

When the weather is bad and you stand out of the rain, in a doorway, with a neighbor who says, "A nasty day, eh?" his words tell you nothing about the state of the world that is not apparent to both of you. Nor are they intended as description: you can see for yourself that it is raining. They do not constitute a request, either—he does not expect you to lend him an umbrella. All he is doing is conveying to you a vague feeling of depression epitomized by the color of the sky. It would be offensive to interpret his comment differently and exclaim, "Sounds to me as though you're depressed this morning, Monsieur Martin." To do any such thing would be intrusive, unless you are close friends. What M. Martin is asking for is just that his discontent be quietly acknowledged. He expects, too, that his ability to share meaning and affect will be supported by reciprocation. Such a reason for speaking is no different from a child's: in the language of children, the determining factors are neither necessity nor the urgency of a need. A child's first words do not express hunger or thirst. They certainly manifest a demand, but it is a demand for shared meaning (and when I say "meaning," it means "affect").

The Main Stages of Language Acquisition in Ordinary Children

Seen from a psychoanalytical perspective, any subject who wishes to speak must be feeling uneasy at being confronted with a changing world and must want to transform but not evacuate the tension being experienced.[1] The very first protosignifiers that are observed conform to this type of situation: the syllables are unstable, but their intonation is clear. The first of these is the intonation of appeal: on a rising melody, it is a marker of the urgency of the child's resorting to another to cope with astonishment and to understand with the support of the other's compassion. Then there is the intonation of surprise: on a falling melody, it is a marker of the fact that the child, though at first destabilized by what he has perceived, is managing to cope with his disturbance unaided, though still in the presence of somebody else.

Even the very earliest stable signifiers spoken by a child (apart from *papa* and *maman*) are not words that mean objects, either. They are words for states of feeling. The *ça* (= "that") that accompanies the child's first pointing at about twelve months old, then the recurring words like *ha* or *voilà* (= "there," "look"), *encore* (= "again"), or *non* (= "no") all belong to the same register: none of these words speaks of a definite aspect of reality; what they do speak of is what the child is feeling through contact with the world, how she is experiencing her own thinking and the presence and thinking of someone else.

Pointing and the Question of Surprise

Pointing is an act of communication on the threshold of speech. It is said to occur at a moment when a child tries to have his mother share something he finds interesting. Seen from the perspective of its construction, it is a complex thing. First, the child will point toward the object that he or she wishes to show. Then, a glance at the mother's eyes will try to bring them toward what is being pointed at. This to-and-fro of hand and eye will be accompanied by a first word, a signifying syllable expressed as *ça* (= "that"), possibly mispronounced but recognizable. This complex gesture will have had precursors, but in its definitive form it will appear between nine and twelve months, an age at which a child has the capacity to construct a shared focus of attention.

---

1. This chapter owes much to the work of Dr. M. Brigaudiot and to the further research we carried out jointly after the completion of her doctoral work. I am glad to record here my gratitude to her. For all matters dealt with in this chapter, see Brigaudiot and Nicolas (1990).

The Object of Joint Attention

What is the child trying to show? Some authors take the view that it is
the thing the child wishes to have, something to eat or a toy just out of
reach: pointing is seen as a kind of aborted snatching movement that turns
into mime as a way of seeking the adult's assistance. Here we have once
more an explanation by need, to which I do not subscribe. A child who
points up at a bird in the sky does not necessarily wish it to be put into
his hand. He is pointing because the flying thing is of interest and especially because he wants to be spoken to about it. Some will say that a
bird is a salient object, but what requires definition is what salience consists of. It might be a black patch on a white wall, a bump on a smooth
surface, anything that makes a shape stand out against a uniform background. I am not convinced that the salience of any object can be reduced to an objective property of it. Nothing is salient per se: it is made
salient by the interest taken in it. In this context, Freudian concepts show
how invaluable they remain: what interests a child is anything that conveys a feeling of disquieting strangeness, whatever brings to mind a
memory without the certainty that what is seen and what is remembered because of what is seen are one and the same thing. This happens, for example, every time the child sets eyes on something that
resembles something familiar but is not quite what is familiar. Or it may
happen when the child is in a familiar context but is faced with an element that is unusual or incongruous. It is at such moments that the child
feels surprise and a disquieting strangeness: he has been expecting to be
faced with something but finds himself faced with something different
(something that he deems "different" by reference to his very expectation of it and by reference to a representation that he expected to be
validated). That, at least, is my interpretation of a child's surprise and
feeling of disquieting strangeness. There is another interpretation, which
sees surprise as a reaction to the fact that, when one has been expecting
nothing, something may happen. In my view, that would be a case of
being simply dumbfounded. To be surprised, one must be in a situation
that first creates an expectation, then fails to meet it. Surprise comes
from the disparity between what is expected and what is discovered.
The object out there that is pointed at, the salient object, is an object
of surprise, an object that brings to mind a memory that is invariably
out of keeping with what is perceived.

Same/Not Same

If that is the case, what does a child mean by pointing at a patch of light on a wall while saying *Ça* (= lit. "that")? First and foremost, it means the child is intrigued or uneasy—intrigued at perceiving something in the real world that recalls a perceptual memory and uneasy because what is perceived does not exactly coincide with the perception as stored in the memory. In part, the child vents and gets rid of the uneasiness by saying *Ça* (= "that") in a movement of exclamation and surprise. But this word is also the mark of an uncertain identification between the present perception and the memorized perception, or rather the mark of a comparative juxtaposition of the two: there is a disparity, but there is also an evocative relation. The feeling of disquieting strangeness comes from the contrastiveness of this link. A child who points and says *Ça* (= "that") is basically saying, "Tell me that what I think is a patch of light like the one you and I saw the other day really does have something to do with a patch of light, even though it may not be the same one." Faced with the discrepancy between the present perception and the memorized record of a perception, the child is asking you to confirm his ability to perceive a connection (though not an equivalence or an exact match) in something he sees to be "different" but "related." If his mother takes the present perception as he takes it, then the exact match may not be possible, and he can cease any attempt at making it. As a result, this perception will become an indicator of a genuine representation. This acceptance of the impossibility of establishing exact sameness between two incidences of a similar perceptible phenomenon can be achieved only if there is somebody in addition to me who remembers here and now the light that was there the other morning when I woke up and it was warm. The stability of the representation, despite the discrepancy between the different objects effectively perceived, and despite the discrepancy between the successive manifestations of the patch of light, is guaranteed by the fact that the subject can think that what reminds him of it in the present situation reminds not only him but also the other person whom he addresses. This is the founding consensual illusion: what I see recalls a thing and that thing it recalls for you, too. Herein lies solace for the impossibility of the exact match; it is this solace that transforms the content, memorized perception, into a representation. This puts an end to the search for an effective identity, point by point, between the image kept by the subject's memory and each realization of it that can be discovered over time in the outside world, since the subject knows that the other person with whom he is looking at the world shares his conviction that, though there is no exact sameness between the sign seen and the representation memorized, nonetheless a link and an equivalence can be made.

Pointing is thus at the confluence of a great many aptitudes. It presupposes the ability not only to imagine that one's gesture has a meaning for the person to whom it is addressed but also to presume the existence of thought in that person. One has to feel able to attract that person's thought for the purpose of focusing it on a particular object. One has to endow that object with the status of a sign (it is not the object that is important but the cluster of thoughts for which it stands as a metonym). In addition, one has to put both information and affect into a single gesture, since pointing means not just looking at an object but also showing, and wanting to share, one's surprise.

A Relation That Underlies a Great Many Symbolic Forms

Between the object actually perceived and the representation it arouses, Ça (= "that") marks a link that is both likeness and unlikeness. This linkage is what underlies a great many symbolic forms. First, it makes possible the organizing of categorization: the object pointed at in the actual dimension is then stored in the same category as the one whose representation was aroused, despite the divergences acknowledged between them (and, besides, not all the elements included in a category are identical). Second, the relation can also lead to the establishment of an approximation: the object perceived in the actual dimension is compared with another, though not really assimilated to the category that the other belongs to; toward the end of this chapter, we shall see a child who says, when confronted by a crab, "like tortoise," thus marking a likeness between the object just discovered and the one he is thinking of, though he does not attempt to assimilate them (a distinction marked by the use of "like"). Or, third, the relation may be the one that links a detail or a circumstance to the event it calls to mind. If, for instance, a child points at a fire extinguisher, it is not in the hope that his mother will identify the object or say its name. What it means is that the child remembers having seen a comparable thing when they went together to get a document from the town hall and is suggesting that his mother should talk about this shared memory.

This explains why a child will say *Ça* (= "that") about a lamp, an arm-chair, a dog, or a frog, using the same unchanging syllable for each different object pointed at. The word does not designate a particular object; it encodes the affective process involved in linking together two poles: the visible element in the present situation and the unactual element present in the memory. And this linking is organized through, and sustained by, a relation with another person, as the child asks the mother to confirm it.

However, pointing and saying *Ça* (= "that") define only a first mode of linkage between a sign and the representation that corresponds to it. For a representation to be fully a representation, it must in addition be freed from the direct stimulus provided by the fortuitous presence of an actual element. It must reach the stage where the restimulation of the other morning's transaction over the patch of light no longer depends on whether or not I see a patch of light in my present situation. This stage is reached between fifteen months and two years, when a child starts to repeat words. In repeating words, the child is playing not with sounds but with sounds that he experiences as variants of representations. In repeating words, the child is playing with images in his head, needing no further stimulation in his present situation than the sound of the words in his ears and the movements of their pronunciation in his mouth. None of this, unlike the patch of light on the wall, is given to him by the outside world. He makes it up.

The Words of Affect

As we have seen, the word *Ça* (= "that") spoken while the child is pointing does not vary from object to object. It describes none of the qualities of the thing itself but says everything about the purpose of the person pointing. The words that emerge soon after this are similar in nature. For example, very often what comes next is *Voilà* (= "Look," "There"), which expresses the child's satisfaction at seeing a project become a reality (a sort of cry of triumph expressing satisfaction at the achieving of an objective, comparable with the adult utterance *Et voilà !* (= "Look at that!" or "There we are!"). Something similar though converse can be seen in *encore* (= "again"), where the child realizes that the present situation differs from what he wants and so utters a wish for a return to the more desirable situation of which he has formed a representation. This entails an anticipatory perspective, involving a mode of temporality called "aspect" in linguistics. Briefly, "aspect" is a way of interpreting the present situation by reference to a representation that can give meaning to it. Saying *encore* (= "again") means having noticed the lack of what is now required once more and wishing that what is about to happen should resemble a situation recently experienced. It is an utterance related to the immediate future tense. It is a way of giving meaning to what one can see by relating it to what one wants. As such, it belongs to the category of words that express a subject's states of feeling, as does, of course, *Non* (= "No"), with its expression of refusal. *Non* expresses no representation but merely indicates that the child is resisting the adult's immediate intention for him. The last words to arise in this series, *apu* (= *il n'y a plus*, "no more," "none left," "all gone") and *fini* (= "finished," "over"), mark the fact that the child acknowledges a state of reality and sees it forlornly as being full of irreparable absence. What is significant here is that the word spoken indicates a new ability of the child's to retain interest in a representation now gone beyond recall.

What is peculiar to all of these utterances (*ça, voilà, encore, non, apu*) is that they are linked to affective events that recur regularly in the child's activity in the world and that they enable expression of what is felt. They are not words for things or definite objects. They are words for emotional states reacting to changes that affect the world. This is presumably why these very first words have often escaped the attention of observers: if one seeks a meaning for them in the world outside the child, it is an unstable one. The only stable meaning for them should be sought inside the subject whose affect and point of view they define.

Onomatopoeias and Motor Activity

It must be stressed, of course, that not all of a child's earliest words express affect or a point of view on representations. There are some that have actual content. These are the ones that correspond to onomatopoeias of the "vroom" or "moo" variety and that figure in connection with a highly particular class of objects: animate beings that are like children themselves in that, though they have no language, they can move and make noises (cars, dogs, cats, cows, and so on). Unlike words that express affect and a point of view, onomatopoeias say something about the world. They do so, however, without designating an object. Initially, an onomatopoeia is an integral part of the scenario involving motor play. An onomatopoeia such as "vroom vroom" is nothing more than a detail of the miming with the toy car adding to the pretense that it is a real car moving and making a noise by itself. Saying "vroom vroom" also requires a certain motor activity of the mouth and phonation apparatus; the signifier, by virtue of this activity entailed in producing it, is thus on the same level as the hand movement needed to push the object along the floor. There is an illusion of referentiality, which is created by the presence of this particular object within the scenario. But the onomatopoeia is first and foremost something spoken as part of a game with an adult, within a ritual of interaction and turn-taking: each of us says "vroom" as we run the car to and fro between us. The word, as a fragment of an interactive scenario, belongs to an exchange. But gradually it will become in addition a word that the subject speaks to himself, self-directed speech.

On the whole, onomatopoeias as signifiers have several effects. First, they foster the making of contrasts related to the nature of the referents. The fact that the child hears the adult say "vroom" while pushing the car will become the thing that marks off play with a car from play with a plastic cow, which they move about while saying "moo." Second, they help the child toward a measure of mastery of the ritual. This is particularly clear-cut in contrast to the *ça, voilà, encore, non, apu* group of utterances, in which language gives the child a way to overcome what affects him by bodying out what he is feeling without necessarily acting upon the world. With onomatopoeias, the child takes an active role in the enacting of the scenario.

In general, onomatopoeias usually develop in four observable stages. In the first of these, an onomatopoeia is associated with an extremely circumscribed context. The child will say "vroom" only if a particular car is used in particular circumstances, for instance, if it is taken out of the toybox in his own room and run across from the bed to the window. He will not say "vroom" with another car or if the car is made to run over the tiled floor of the kitchen. Nor will he say "vroom" if he merely points at the car, not wanting to play with it but just to show it. There are some children who never go beyond this stage. Much more usually, however, there is a development in the direction of generalization: anything that can play the part of the car in a given scenario will be said to be "vroom," anything that can roll, such as a bobbin or a spool. On this point, the specialized literature speaks of overextension, but it seems the process is not exactly that. In fact, at this stage the child manages to abstract from the play situation a particular feature; every time this feature reappears, even in situations that are very different, he will mark the coincidence by saying "vroom." "Vroom" is an indication of only a partial commonality and not of absolute identity between the situations. Also, when the initial situation is complex, the child may vary the indicator; and "vroom" may become not just things that can roll but even things that may resemble a little box into which one can fit other things, as into the little car. The fact remains, though, that "vroom" will be used solely in connection with a scenario that involves motor activity, for anything that can roll like a little car or anything that can have things put into it. The toy car will not be "vroom" if the child merely points at it but does not play with it, any more than the family car that he sits in will be. What determines the use of the onomatopoeia in different situations requiring different objects is the unchanging fact that it belongs in a motor activity scenario.

Joining Up

The question of how the child comes to generalize the use of a word like "vroom," extending it first to play with the same car in different situations, then to different cars, then to any object with wheels, is an interesting one. The process relies essentially on the ability to compare two situations that are not identical in everything so as to define a relation between what is present in the here and now and what has been memorized. The source of the linkage may lie as much in the nature of the objects as in the pleasure that the child brings to bear upon them.

This period of generalization is a decisive stage. It presumably arises from the fact that the two initial lines of linguistic productions—the one encoding affect (*ça*, *voilà*, *encore*, *non*, *apu*) and the one encoding motor activity (onomatopoeias)—reach a point where they join up. One and the same word may be usable in several dimensions. So "vroom" may no longer designate just a turn-taking motor activity scenario organized around an object: the child may take to using the term while pointing at the toy car, for instance, if he sees it in an unexpected place. That is, this term will take on the role initially allotted to *ça ?* (= "that"), but only in the restricted context relating to the toy car. It is then and only then that the term comes to have a properly referential status. "Vroom" is no longer an order meaning "I want us to start playing cars." It is a signifier and has a signified. This means that play with representations via manipulation of the signifier can now develop.

The Beginnings of Grammar

Once a word like "vroom" comes to be used not just as an invitation to play with a car, the term is available for incorporation into a combinatory system which is grammar. For this to happen, it need only be combined with intonation: "vroom!" spoken with an imperative tone (a strong falling intonation) expresses the desire to be handed a toy car that is out of reach; and "vroom?" will be used interrogatively of a toy tank, because it looks rather like a car, although its turret and gun also make it look different. Once the referential word bespeaks a representation and not a plan of action, its intonation (which may mark, for example, the distinction between an order and an inquiry) can incorporate it into the combinatory system of grammar, long before any grammatical inflexions have been learned.

Classifying

As soon as a word like "vroom" stops being a potential act, one begins to see the appearance of spontaneous classifying and differentiating procedures, suggesting that the child's aim is to clarify what distinguishes two comparable objects. Manipulation of the representation of things takes the place of manipulation of the things themselves. This is also the time when it becomes easier for an adult to correct the child's errors. It is about this time too that the child starts taking pleasure in repeating words: repeating a word becomes a way of playing with its representation via its signifier. It is probably this that prepares what is commonly called the "vocabulary explosion," about the end of the second year. At this stage, the child tries to regularize his or her use of words by making clear distinctions between categories of comparable objects.

Comparison

In connection with the regularization of referential vocabulary, I cannot resist the urge to tell a story about a child without language disorder. At the age of eighteen months, on a beach, he saw a strange animal coming out of the water. He looked at his mother and, by gesture and expression, turning his hands upward and with his mouth in an O-shape, he showed incredulity, astonishment, even slight dismay. His whole posture could have been translated as: "What sort of an animal might that be?" His mother, aware of what he was feeling, told him it was a *crabe* (= "crab"). He tried to repeat *crabe* but could not manage it, defeated by the consonant cluster *cr*. So he shook his head and said simply, "Like tortoise."

The initial cause of the child's astonishment was no doubt the similarity that he noticed between what he could see and something he already knew, a tortoise. He was aware that crabs and tortoises had some things in common, both being crawling animals with a shell. But he was also aware that they were not the same animal: one of them had feet and the other one had claws; one of them came out of the sea and the other one was to be seen in gardens. In his frustration at not being able to reproduce the proper signifier, he fell back on his original assessment, which was a comparison of the crab with a tortoise. However, whatever differences he had noted between them had been corroborated by his mother's word: there was a relation from one to the other, but one was not the other. This explains his decisive recourse to "like," which is a way of marking the presence in the signifier of a relation, a link, a commonality without exact sameness. "Like" means something is both similar and not similar. This child had reached a level of symbolization at which he could recognize that something could resemble something else without being exactly the same in all respects. He had progressed from the logic of categories to the logic of approximation. In the logic of categories, any individual can either be a tortoise or not be a tortoise, but there is nothing in between; whereas in the logic of approximation, an animal can be "like a tortoise" without actually becoming one. This approach fosters the making of a link between two things that one nonetheless contrives to keep distinct from each other.

Two Years, Two Words

Language gradually becomes established at the intersection of all the axes involving a subject's symbolization: relation to others, relation to the content of his or her own thinking, affect, motor activity, automatic speech, intentional speech. Words are no longer restricted to a single use. Then, about the age of two, as the "vocabulary explosion" is happening, there is a second achievement: statements of two words. As has often been pointed out, this is the time when the child can dispense with the support of the present situation and engage in the elaboration of a common theme with an adult: if there are two terms, the first of them can establish the topic, while the second can provide the comment. In reality, however, the earliest such statements often follow a different pattern. First there are sequences composed of separate words, each of which is a reformulation of the previous one. Then gradually there develops an intonation melody that unifies all the elements of a sequence, giving it the structure of a proper statement. When a child starts to say things like "Give that car there," such a statement is made of three successive elements ("Give," "that car," and "there"), each of which develops the preceding one (basically putting into words the acts of pointing and reaching for the object). Later, when two words make a single statement, the child puts his comment into the one he speaks first (his point of view, for example, on a matter of disagreement) and the topic it refers to into the second one. A child being spoonfed by his mother but wanting to feed himself will say, "Me eat." With this pairing of words, even though essential skills remain to be acquired (the ability to use "I," to tell stories, to make comparisons), the basics of the symbolic operations expressed through the use of language are now in place.

12

From Sense to Sound and Back Again

I have just outlined the principal stages in the acquisition of language from the perspective of symbolization. Here I want to stress certain essentials in the grounding of language as a mechanism that brings together sound and sense. This chapter therefore deals with language as an instrument of production and recognition of speech. In children who are "merely" dysphasic, this dimension of language is particularly underdeveloped.

Generally speaking, to be capable of communicating and speaking, human beings must be able to divide what is said to them into sequences of identifiable and comprehensible signifiers. They must also be able to mobilize sufficient energy to produce words out of the ideas they have, while having in addition the ability to make the mouth and phonation apparatus perform the actions required to utter these words in the proper order. There is, of course, a long tradition of speculative attempts to explain the neuropsychological processes that underlie these movements of encoding and decoding, which it is not my purpose to rehearse here. All I propose to do, as in the chapter on symbolization, is to highlight several elements crucial to the difficulties of dysphasic children. In so doing, I show something of the influence and effects of the neurological mechanism (what Freud called the "speech apparatus") on the process of symbolization as a whole.

The First Months of Life

The work of Jacques Mehler in particular has established that, from the earliest days of extrauterine life, children have the ability not only to differentiate syllables and recognize phonemes but also to recognize patterns of intonation (Mehler & Dupoux 1990). To begin with, however, what they perceive does not seem to have a bearing on what they produce. It is not until about the age of eight months that the lallations they make in the cradle are composed solely of the phonemes of the language they are hearing. From an instrumental point of view, it might be thought that this production has been informed by their perception. But, looking at the emergence of this standard babbling from the point of view of the evolution of the psyche, René Diatkine makes the point that from the age of eight months the child trying to speak identifies with his mother speaking to him. This idea coincides with the fact that it is approximately at this age that the child's representation of the mother stabilizes. If she is approaching the bedroom where he is, he is capable of knowing this in advance by giving meaning to the sounds that precede her appearance; this ability derives from the fact that he has made a representation of the mother that he can draw on to make sense of what he is hearing before she comes into sight. This idea can also help us interpret the fear shown by a child of that age when a stranger tries to play with him: the stranger's play recalls the representation of his mother, yet his perception of the strange person does not correspond to the image he has of her. Hence his anxiety.

So, by about eight months, an important change has happened; both the production of phonemes and intonation are affected. Chronologically, there is a first phase when the child seems to use his voice to explore all sorts of intonations, then another phase when his changes of pitch approximate better the intonations of the adult, especially when he is addressing someone (though if he is talking to himself, the modulations are less marked). So his intonation will rise with an inquiry or an appeal to someone else but will fall when he is talking to himself or expressing surprise at, say, a discovery.

Two Modes of Energy

Once phonemes and intonation are established, a child can acquire the use of early language. This takes place at about twelve months, by which time the child possesses approximately twenty words, some of which are linked to emotion and affect and define the child's point of view on things and others (such as animal noises) refer to objects and beings in the outside world. In fact, at that age, when a child wants to say something, one of two things happens: either she reproduces the general tune of a statement while giving an inaccurate pronunciation of the actual syllables (she knows the song but not the words) or else she focuses her effort on the principal consonant of the essential word and tries to reproduce it as best she can. In my view, this dichotomy confirms the hypothesis of the two modes of energy required for speech: the children who retain the tune are using only a memory linked to feeling, whereas those who put their effort into the principal consonant are focused on motor activity and the act of phonation (Boysson-Bardies 1996). In time, children gradually develop both of these modes.

It has been known since Freud and Jackson that whichever type of energy is mobilized—affect or motor activity—each of them also has two distinct circuits, one of them short, the other long: an "automatic" circuit and an "intentional" circuit (Jackson 1931). Swearing functions through the automatic, and the formulation of any complex idea through the intentional. I propose to begin by clarifying that distinction.

Automatic Speech

Automatic speech is a type of reflex utterance produced in reaction to a particular situation. It is a mode of speech that requires a high level of energy and results in a limited number of relatively unvarying expressions. In automatic speech related to emotion, we find, for example, swearing and exclamations of surprise. Neither of these ways of speaking draws on representation. A blurt of speech is the subject's all but involuntary resolution of his or her predicament. As well as such automatic verbalizations related to emotion, there are others linked to motor activity, for instance the words uttered as part of a sociability ritual, such as the "Good-bye" that accompanies a handshake and the opening of a door. Though such a moment of leave-taking may be an emotional one and the role of affect in it is undoubtedly not negligible, the actual articulation of "Good-bye" is an integral part of the motor ritual of grasping a hand and opening a door. What stimulates the speech movement is the situation with its linked sequence of actions. Here, as with swearing, no meaning preexists in the mind of the speaker, and the production of language is equally automatic.

Intentional Speech

Intentional speech is another way of speaking altogether. Here, it is not the situation that brings out the word: the word arises out of, and is preceded by, thinking. For thought to be capable of setting in motion the words that can express it, what is required—this, at any rate, is my hypothesis—is that the speaking of them, the speaker's starting up of his or her articulatory movement, should have become a sort of fictitious actualization of the motor project or emotion originally linked to the situation denoted by them. When such is the case, it is not that an emotion or a motor scenario activates a word but rather that the word's articulation corresponds to an affective or motor outburst. Intentional speech "converts" a thought into words. The energy to be mobilized arises from that representation. A child who thinks of her teddy will transfer the pleasure and affection associated with the toy onto the word "teddy." If the object is not present, she will fall back on saying the word, taking from its phonation something of the pleasure that handling the toy would afford her. The pleasure connected to the representation is communicated to the spoken word, and therein lies the source of the energy essential to its utterance. In other words, in the earliest days of automatic speech, when the child is overcome by an affect (surprise, rejection, or whatever), the very act of saying this or that word is a way of venting the feeling. As time goes on, however, this relation is inverted; when speech becomes intentional, it is by saying the word that the child comes to have the feeling. No longer does this or that signifier express surprise, refusal, desire, triumph, disappointment; it is speaking the appropriate word that connotes the sensation of surprise, refusal, desire, triumph, disappointment. At the same time, the distinctions that mark each of these sensations become more marked and more stable, as the difference between signifiers such as *encore*, *voilà*, *non*, and *apu* helps the child become better at managing the affective signifieds that correspond to each of them.

On the motor side, an analogous development is noticeable. It can be seen in what becomes, for instance, of a signifier linked to motor activity, an onomatopoeia such as "vroom," initially an integral part of a motor scenario involving a toy car. The speaking of the word is a set of actions belonging to the game. But, gradually, the totality of the scenario, from the saying of the word to the hand movement, becomes concentrated in the speaking of the onomatopoeia: the rolling of the *r* in "vroom" eventually comes to crystallize the complete idea of turning motion associated with the vehicle and its wheels. From this point on, as the idea of the car now stimulates the idea of something that runs along, it becomes possible to organize the intentional circuit of speech. The idea of something that runs along is inchoately actualized in the child's saying the signifier *r*. The notion of the car activates the energy required to say "vroom."

In automatic speech, the situation directly mobilizes the affect or the motor activity that sends the words out of the mouth. There is no mediation through thought. However, when the pronouncing of a word can crystallize through displacement the act or affect attached to the thing, thinking of the thing is enough to activate the energy required to utter the word. When one cannot act upon the thing, the mouth can magically conjure it. The energy necessary to speech derives from this fictitious actualization and speech becomes intentional.

A child's first register of speech is obviously automatic, and he has no access to the dimension of intentional speech until the diverse modes of automatic speech have had time to link up. It is this mingling of automatic ways of speaking that enables intentional speech to take off. Moreover, it frequently happens that, when a child with a disorder does eventually manage to make an effort at deliberate verbalization, once his utterances have ceased being the mere automatic outcome of a situation in the here and now, or when what he says runs to more than a single word, the quality of both voice and delivery changes. Sometimes a note of hoarseness creeps in or the elocution becomes forced, as though rote learned. The reason for this is not that the lengthening of the utterances overtaxes the memory. It is, rather, the fact that saying more than a single word about a situation presupposes that one is able to make sense of it from different perspectives and to juggle these perspectives without each of them canceling out the one before. The difficulty lies in the fact of speaking while thinking, because one must keep changing one's point of view on the things one is trying to say.

During the phase of automatic speech, what the subject does or feels serves as the direct basis of whatever he says. Of necessity, this directness induces a putting into words with no possibility of paraphrase. When language becomes intentional, things can be put into words through recourse to thought, and thought itself can thus be clarified.

Intentional Speech and Thought

Generally, the displacement I have been referring to is responsible for what psychoanalysts call the economic effect of language. This describes the fact that, by putting something into words, one can reduce tension in the psychic apparatus without completely annulling it. What happens is roughly as follows: whenever one experiences a discrepancy between desire and reality, one's psyche is subject to tensions. The simplest way to counter the resulting state of dissatisfaction is to vent it in movement, thus annulling the tensions. This makes for total quietude, but, in order to think, there must actually be some residue of tension left in the psychic apparatus, since thinking means transforming a tension that is tolerable. This is what intentional speech contrives to do. On the one hand, as speaking a word is a magic action done to the thing denoted by it, speech helps reduce psychic tension; on the other, as the movement is limited, the reduction is only relative and the tension continues. The signified of a word links the tension to a representation.

There are children who, though they have automatic language (at the level of exclamations and onomatopoeias), cannot proceed to intentional speech. Often, their speaking of a word is a mere motor discharge, without the slightest association with thought content. For this state of affairs to change, such children must become able to reestablish a representation content in relation to the words they use, even if these are only onomatopoeias or exclamations. By way of helping them to put representation into the language circuit, one can simply repeat any of their spontaneous exclamations, because once an exclamation is uttered by somebody else it ceases to be a mere discharge and becomes a representation of affect. Repeating what a child says is a way of proving to him that one can think about what he is thinking about when he speaks a signifier. It is a way of restoring the signifier's signified, which is, as it were, erased in automatic speech, where the word's only function is as a spoken sound that makes for a reduction of tension.

Organizing the Mental Lexicon: Common Terms,
Proper Names, Grammatical Markers

It is obvious that formulation of thought depends on the storing of words in the head, that is to say, on the making of what is sometimes called a "mental lexicon." These days, it is believed that the organizing of this lexicon goes through different stages during a child's development.

There is a long period during which meaning is what determines the structuring of the lexicon. Signifiers that correspond to a particular area of activity attract one another and form networks: "spade" connects to "rake" and "castle" to "sand," and so on. Some associations are based on similarities of the impressions conveyed by the signifiers: "honey" and "sunshine," "warm" and "nice." Then, when the lexicon reaches about fifty words, a change occurs. This can be seen through a study of the mistakes of pronunciation made by children who have no language problem. Up to fifty words, they make relatively few mispronunciations, although they do reduce words that are too long to their first or last syllable. Then, when the lexicon contains fifty words or more, though they get the number of syllables right, they start introducing systematic simplifications: a word like *lapin* (= "rabbit"), formerly pronounced *pin*, suddenly becomes *papin*. Such mispronunciations are so systematic that they can be simulated by computer. What explains this phenomenon is that, beyond a certain point, memory is saturated and requires a reorganization of the whole system. To accommodate the signifiers, the brain no longer stores them in a single mass. For each word, it compiles a set of instructions: first, the number of syllables; then the main consonant (the one that gives the shape of the root) and its place in the whole word; then the value of the other consonants (preceding or following); last, the coloring of the vowels. The consonants, as an ordered unit, structure the skeleton of a word. In a spoken statement, it is this consonantal skeleton that serves to make a word identifiable to the ear. Each set of instructions serves to reconstruct each word required. So, every time one wants to pronounce a word, one first recomputes it. This is exactly the sequence of stages we go through when having trouble finding a word that we have "on the tip of our tongue": we remember first how many syllables it has, then a main consonant, and suddenly we can grasp the whole word. This also explains why a child will start saying *papin* instead of *lapin* at the very moment when his vocabulary is restructuring. In fact, he is starting to use the sets of instructions, which has the immediate effect of making it more difficult to pronounce any given word. So he starts to stumble on words that he used not to stumble on, remembering that the instructions stipulate two syllables, the second of which starts with *p*, but forgetting the rest, which makes him put the same consonant at the beginning of the first syllable.

The advantage of the new organization is that it gives much faster access to the words of the lexicon, because of the ordering inside each "area of meaning" on the basis of the number of syllables and the value of the main consonant. However, the disadvantage of it is that the signifier of a stored word has to be recomputed. The search for a word now brings up not a signifier ready for use but a whole bundle of information that has to be properly reconfigured before one can start speaking. This is where children go wrong.

Mispronunciations of this type are, of course, not nearly of the same order of gravity as what can happen when the reorganization of the mental lexicon does not occur. The only option a child can then fall back on is that provided by the meanings of words. This makes the search for a word very complicated; by way of simplification, the child will curtail his different lexical networks so as to use a single salient word for all purposes. He will say "knife" when what he means is not only a knife but a fork or a spoon. He will never mix up the real objects so named, but, for talking about any sort of cutlery, he has only one word.

The Arrangement of Words in the Mental Lexicon

On the whole, once a child has a mental lexicon of more than fifty words, it can be assumed that its structuring tends to be the same as an adult's. It comprises three areas, each of which corresponds to elements that are activated in different ways. The first consists of all the elements of the lexicon other than proper names; the second contains proper names; and the third is composed of grammatical elements (articles, prepositions, inflexions, and derivations). Each of these three sorts of words behaves differently when one is trying to remember them, repeating them, or reading them. Nor do they necessarily represent identical difficulties for aphasic patients. Common terms (common nouns, verbs, adjectives, adverbs) are implicated in more than one network, every common noun for example belonging to a particular family but perhaps figuring also in various set expressions. In addition, it belongs to a particular area of practice, one that can produce different metaphorical organizations. A word such as *œil* (= "eye"), for instance, is manifestly a member of the family *œil, œillade, œillet, œilleton* (= "eye," "eyeing," "eyelet," "eyepiece"), while figuring in expressions as different as *œil-de-bœuf* (= "bull's-eye window") and *faire de l'œil à quelqu'un* (= "to give someone the eye"). But it also belongs to the area of practice associating *œil-pupille-lunettes* ("eye-pupil-glasses"). And, in addition, it is the metaphorical nucleus that gives expression to ideas of close attachment or great value, like "the apple of one's eye" (= *tenir à quelque chose comme à la prunelle de ses yeux*) or "costing the earth" (= *coûter un œil*). Sometimes, too, a link may be made between the pronouncing of a word and certain aspects of its meaning, as in the *r* of onomatopoeias like *broum* (= "vroom") or other words expressive of rotation.

The Areas of the Mental Lexicon

When trying to put into words an idea to be expressed intentionally, one first seeks out the motor program that corresponds to the essential signifier in whatever one wants to say. The starting up of the speech apparatus will be caused by an action or an affect linked to the referent that corresponds to the object or action one wants to allude to. This is what gives the initial impetus that activates the different networks within which the required signifier is stored. Its motor program is then preactivated, and it can be brought into action. The more a word is fraught with affect or the more easily its referent can be manipulated, the more readily its starting-up energy can be mobilized. In other words, the easier it is to find the corresponding word. This can be observed in patients who have trouble finding their words. If they are asked to put names to pictures of concrete objects, they find it easier to think of the word for a hammer (*un marteau*) or a fork (*une fourchette*) than words like *arbre* (= "tree"), *nuage* (= "cloud"), or *soleil* (= "sun"). Comparable in their affective qualities, the objects that correspond to the words "hammer" (*marteau*) and "fork" (*fourchette*) are more easily manipulated than the objects that correspond to "tree" (= *arbre*) and "sun" (= *soleil*). Abstract words are also easily manipulated. Geometric figures such as circles, squares, or triangles are abstractions; but they are also shapes whose contours are made by definite hand motions, which explains why some patients should find it easier to think of the word *carré* (= "square") than of the word *arbre* (= "tree").

Further, every common noun is associated with a minimal syntactic structure that determines how it can participate in a statement (the type of words that must both precede and follow it). This promotes the search for the words to surround the central word in the definitive utterance.

This, roughly, is what is entailed in the structuring and the implementing of words that belong to the common vocabulary.

Proper Nouns and Grammar Words

It is not my purpose here to hazard a definition of the special status en-joyed by proper nouns that sets them apart from common nouns. I shall say merely that it is much easier to forget a proper noun than a common noun and that the system of various networks (word families, for instance, or set expressions) does not exist for proper nouns, which is presumably why they are more difficult to grasp. Needless to say, such a sketchy de-scription is inadequate, if only because there is a difference in incidence and in extent between forgetting people's first names and forgetting proper nouns.

As for grammar words, those morphological elements that are required for signifiers to figure in an utterance, no one ever has any trouble locat-ing them: at a loss for words we may be, unable to remember a turn of phrase, but we are never at a loss for prepositions, articles, or grammati-cal endings. Grammar words, in their encoding, do not have the same status as other words. This difference in status between lexical words and grammar words is confirmed by people who have difficulties in reading aloud, such as a German patient who found it impossible to read gram-mar words in her own language: "Here's another of those nasty little words," she would say when faced with the word *es* (= "it"), though she had no difficulty in reading a lexical word containing the same number of letters, *Ei* (= "egg") (Bierwisch & Weigl 1970). What is striking in this case is not just the difference between reading full words and grammati-cal words; it is the way the patient deduces from *es* that she is dealing with a grammar word, even though her solution to the problem it posed was inappropriate. It gives another reason for supposing that syntax words and lexical words receive different processing. Lexical words are associated with meaning; syntax words have no meaning. Lexical words are very nu-merous; syntax words are finite in number. Lexical words are activated through the circuit of intentional speech, which starts from meaning, func-tions through engaging with affect and motor activity, and subactivates networks of interlinking signifiers that eventually lead to a switching on of the motor skills in the mouth and phonation apparatus; syntactical words, on the other hand, do not function like that. In reading, for example, with any word that has no meaning, differences instantly start to appear; real words are read in a way that is not at all the way in which invented words (like *tivu* or *glapion*) are read. The circuits used to read *garçon* (= "boy") and something meaningless like *glapion* are distinct from each other. One can even induce changes of circuit, as in the following example drawn from my own experience. A man suffering from severe Broca's aphasia found it impossible to read made-up words (like *tivu* or *glapion*), though he had no problem with real words such as *garçon* (= "boy"). However, if *glapion* was put into a syntactical context that gave an illusion of a possible range of meanings, then he could read the word. That is, he was unable to read *tivu* or *glapion* if they stood by themselves in the middle of an otherwise blank page; yet he could read them if they were part of a statement like "Where have you put the tivus?" or "Put those glapions back where you got them immediately." A full explanation of this phenomenon would be too long for inclusion here. Suffice it to say that it shows there are two ways of reading words: the method of deciphering letter by letter and the method of whole-word recognition. Even the latter, of course, starts from the recognition of individual details, which suggest possible readings as the eye travels until the choice is made through reference to the context and the word is pronounced. This works, however, only if the reader suspects that the word in question has a meaning and that it functions within various networks. That is why one can work the illusion of inserting a nonexistent word into a context where it can take on a semblance of meaning: because the reader has the feeling that it might be a genuine lexical word, it is read like one.

The Consonantal Skeleton

I have just discussed the difference between words that exist and words that do not exist, and how one of the latter can be made to become one of the former. I have also been assuming that the signifiers of words that exist also belong to various networks (e.g., families of words, set expressions, metonymic and metaphorical associations, antonyms, synonyms). The links between these different networks, all intersecting at the signifier, must be supported by at least one common material element. In Semitic languages, for instance, such common elements are quite simply the consonants that are the root of a word, forming what I call its consonantal skeleton. This skeleton lies somewhere between the sound of a word and its meaning, though it does not give direct access to either. In fact, it enables us to recognize a sequence of syllables as making a word from our lexicon, even before we have deduced what it must mean. In some cases of Wernicke's aphasia, patients have great difficulty putting a name to objects that they recognize perfectly well. It might be thought that they are incapable of producing the actions required to pronounce the word in question, whereas in fact what is missing is the whole motor program. Faced with the picture of an object for which they cannot find the signifier, they will proceed by trial and error, making tentative approximations. Often, when one of these stabs in the dark actually produces the right word, they will not even notice it but go on trying other ones. This might make one assume there is something wrong with their hearing or that they do not realize what they are saying. Despite this, the same patients are capable not only of correctly repeating genuine words but of reeling off whole sequences of meaningless syllables. If they can do this, it means they have not lost the ability to make the movements corresponding to a syllable spoken and overheard; therefore, their problem does not lie in the area of feedback. What is missing is what Charcot called "the idea of the word" (translated into German by Freud as *Wortvorstellung*). It is this link, whose signifying function is embodied, in my view, in the consonantal skeleton, that ensures the overall identity of a word even before its meaning is mobilized. To recognize the consonantal skeleton of a word is to "feel" that the signifier corresponding to it is linked to several different networks. This "feeling" is what gives a subject the guarantee that a particular word belongs to his or her lexicon; it is a separate thing from the grasping of its meaning.

Formulation of Thought

Having just given a broad-brush account of certain hypotheses about the organization of the mental lexicon, I propose now to present others that deal with the decoding and encoding of meaning. Like the previous ones, these ideas derive in part from my reading on the subject and in part from my reflecting upon some striking clinical encounters.

How does shapeless thinking turn into a completed statement? Spoken discourse, with all its hesitations, makes it manifest that speaking, putting something into words, cannot be done without a certain amount of hard work. There are several stages. First, one must have some notion about which area of meaning is relevant to what one wishes to express; then one must find the word to form the core of the utterance. Next, any words to be associated with this central term have to fit without doing violence to the grammar of the whole. So one has to locate the words required, and, in addition, one must be able to replace this or that word by a synonym so as to keep the syntax coherent. Several models have been devised with the aim of simulating what happens, the most straightforward of which is Garrett's (Garrett 1975). A simple example shows how it works: after a dinner, I offer a lift home to a friend; on the sidewalk he sees me hesitate; then I remember I left my car in a nearby parking lot; I point in its general direction and say, "I left the car in a parking lot just around the corner." To model the way this information gets put into words, the basic premise is that it started as the most imprecise of ideas: an intention to locate an object. This purpose and my gesture emerged simultaneously. At that stage, I had only a general intimation of what I wanted to say. Then I remembered where I had left the car; and I wanted to pass on this information to my friend. In the next stage, I had to divide my imprecise idea into areas of meaning, one of them corresponding to the topic of the object required to be found (my car) and the other to the additional information that I intended to provide (where it was situated in the adjacent parking lot). At this stage, for alluding to the topic of the car, I did not yet know whether I was going to use the word *voiture* (= "car") or perhaps the more familiar *bagnole* (= "jalopy"); to express the position of the car, I did not know whether I was going to say "nearby" or "parking lot." I had chosen neither the words nor even the nature of the words (noun, verb, adverb), though possible words were now emerging. The following stage entailed selecting the signifiers and choosing a structure to accommodate them. After that, I had to make sure the words chosen went in their rightful places. Only then could the production of each detail of the chain in the form of a phoneme get under way.

Understanding the Spoken Word

A question that needs to be asked here is: how do we understand what is said to us? When we listen to a sequence of things said, our first task is to abstract from them the important terms, those that convey the gist, and to arrive at the signified by locating in our own lexicon signifiers identical to those just heard.

If this task had to be carried out the way one looks for a unfamiliar word in a written text, it would take a very long time; and that is not our method for understanding the spoken word. First, the physical setting of the dialogue generally gives us an initial idea of what the other speaker is going to say; second, what we have already gleaned from things just said can give a focus to our hypotheses and bias us toward expectation of certain signifiers that might be used. Eventually, there comes a moment when we must recognize the meaning of the words we are hearing. This can happen only through a dividing up of the chain of sound. Here, intonation is of the first importance: in French, variations in pitch make it possible to localize both the sequence that contains the speaker's topic (or the theme) and the sequence that adds the comment or information. Also, in both of these sequences, differences of pitch make it possible to localize the lexical words, which, in ordinary unemphatic speech, are usually pronounced with higher pitch than the grammatical words. And certain recurring grammatical words (articles, pronouns, auxiliary verbs) suggest the way the whole utterance is organized. For example, after *je* (= "I"), what is expected is a verb; this gives a first clue to the syntactical structure of the ensuing statement. However, once all that has happened, once the scope for searching has been narrowed down by the physical context, the area of meaning, and the grammatical elements, how is the definitive identification of a signifier achieved? Certainly not the way one looks up a word in a dictionary: in the mental lexicon, there is no such thing as alphabetical order. What there is, though, is families of words that have a common consonantal skeleton and form a cluster around the same core of meaning, for example, *boulanger, boulangère,* and *boulangerie* ("baker," "baker's wife," "bakery"), whose skeleton is made from *b, l,* and *g* and that belong to the same family. This is the point at which the final stage of identification begins. When one hears a sequence that one knows is a separate unit of thought, containing a signifier (when one has made the proper word divisions in a sound chain like *Les vautours nichent dans les branches* [= "Vultures nest in the branches"], thereby disambiguating potential but meaningless fragments such as *toursniche* = "turesnest"), one activates the search for the skeletons of words. As consonants are pronounced among the higher notes, which marks them off clearly from the other sounds pronounced among the lower, the discovery of the consonantal skeleton of the required signifier can be achieved without delay. Reverting to the example of *boulangerie,* we can say that when one hears this word, when one is sure it is a signifier though unsure as yet of the meaning of the word or what it corresponds to, it is the three consonants *b, l,* and *g* (the skeleton), which one notices very quickly inside the sequence, that focus our attention on the *boulanger-boulangère-boulangerie* family. This acknowledgment that the sequence heard belongs to that family amounts to the activation of the three terms inside the mental lexicon. Then, so as to identify positively the word heard (to be sure it was *boulangerie* and not *boulangère*), the addressee makes supplementary cross-checks, syllable by syllable.

All the foregoing is obviously an extreme simplification. Nevertheless, it may serve to clarify some references or comments made in the first two parts of this book.

13

Cognitive Implications

A person's way of experiencing the outside world has a bearing on his or her communication and language. This may in turn affect the ways in which the objects of thought to be deployed are separated from one another and constructed. It may also have an effect not only on the signs (whether linguistic or nonlinguistic) that a speaker can construct during an exchange but on the representation he or she may have of an interlocutor.

In this chapter, I want to give a brief reappraisal of some of the areas where children's difficulties seem to arise. The fact is that the cognitive domain, implicated though it is, seems to be neglected by the standard nosographical classifications of dysphasia, with their dichotomy between communication difficulty (allegedly a disorder of psychology and relationships) and language disorder (attributed to a defect in the neurological apparatus that controls production and understanding of speech). In my view, however, there is a third type of disorder, which manifests itself in malfunctions of the nonlinguistic cognitive register and which is quite separate, as I say, from disorders of any strictly aphasiological kind or disorders of relationships. This third type does not bear directly on verbalization but affects the preexisting representations. Using established principles of cognitive science as well as some older psychological ideas deriving from Piaget, one can define the way in which perception and automatic responses to the outside world can influence not only the conditions of communication but also the conceptions and categories that underlie the development of language.

Modularity

The past twenty years or so have seen the development of a theory within cognitive science that posits the workings of perception as the functioning of separate modules, each of which independently processes fragmentary data from the real world (Fodor 1983). This idea sees the interaction of a subject with the world as being based on a set of autonomous routines that, by virtue of their simultaneous processing, can produce extremely rapid automatic reactions to the fluctuations in external stimuli. At a second stage, clearly posterior to the functioning of the modules, central processes start to make genuine representations and to form knowledge that can serve as a focus of attention and finally be put into words. This means that, at the basic module stage, representation, in the sense given to this term in psychology, does not yet exist.

The point of view thus offered by cognitive science on perception is a departure from an accepted norm. It reminds us that the eye is not a photographic plate, nor the ear a magnetic tape: what we perceive of the world does not instantly become an image, a representation. The processing done by the senses brings into play sensors whose measurements are processed independently by separate modules. Each sensor reacts to a certain quality or level of intensity of the stimulus in the dimension corresponding to it. The data gathered can induce reactions in a subject even in the absence of any representation of what the subject is confronted with—the threatening tone of voice of a criminal, for example, can intimidate his victim, even though such a reaction may be unaccompanied by any particular representation. Only at the second stage, when the data receive the central processing, are they associated with a genuine representation of the world. Reverting to the example of eyesight, we can say that visual perception should be considered as a conjunction of specialized modules each of which treats a particular type of information: in an object of perception, color, shape, and movement are all processed separately. Further, each type of information corresponds to a type of cell.

Intermodality

Each sensor, however, may record identical separate measurements in radically different fields. The real value of any such measurement is obviously dependent on the field in which it has been made. In the example of eyesight, and of color in particular, it is commonplace to see gray on an elephant, but not on a wild strawberry. So, for a measurement to be useful, one must be able to form rapid hypotheses about the type of object from which it derives. One can do this only by seeing it as a form and imagining what content it might have. This requires, even before one can have a general interpretation about the object, putting together clues that derive from completely different modules. "Intermodality" is the term given to this activity in cognitive science. It is through intermodality that a subject can locate the domain of an object of perception, by collating clues from heterogeneous processing routines. If, for example, when trying to make out the face of a famous man from a waxwork figure of him, you rely solely on visual information, it will probably take a long time, whereas, if you include also the fact that the original can also speak and move, you will succeed much sooner. However, the second procedure, which entails instantaneously seeing the real face as a living thing, requires the ability to link data from the module for the perception of unmoving shapes to data from the perception of movement and then to combine all of this with the perception of speech. Some of these modules (for instance, the processing of speech and the processing of unchanging shapes) have no inherent connection with one another. Their only way of relating is through the object to be identified.

Once the domain to which an object belongs is identified with certainty, the discriminatory power of the clues one can pick up from it is considerably reinforced. This explains how a baby can have very highly developed discriminatory abilities when dealing with data related to human faces. It has been established, for example, that if babies are shown talking films, they like those with proper synchronization of speech and lip movements better than those without. And, yet, babies do not "see" very well. Their incongruous achievements in this area are made possible by the fact that they "know" that all the data they are working on belong to the domain of the human face. An awareness of the range of meaning within which a visual clue belongs gives such a clue increased discriminability. As we have seen, though, any definition of the range of meaning as such requires the subject to be able to collate data from heterogeneous modules. For a baby to be aware of synchrony between lip movements and spoken words, she must be able to correlate the movements with what she is hearing, which means she must have the potential capacity to connect the module that processes visual data related to movement to the module that processes speech. In a way, intermodality is a corollary of modularity. Modularity posits that the sense organs receive quite separate inputs, each of which is treated independently of the others. Since the meaning of an input depends on the domain from which it derives, what must be quickly identified is the nature of this domain. Intermodality does this by linking data that, though processed in heterogeneous modules, all derive from the same object. Once the domain to which an object belongs has been identified, the potential meanings of any input are reduced, thereby increasing its power of differentiation.

This twofold arrangement of modularity with intermodality guarantees cooperation between modules that nonetheless function in relative isolation from each other. It also facilitates the adoption of a perception strategy based on the nature of the object of perception, rather than on the main sense used in apprehending it, which means that, to recognize a face, one is not going to exploit the same routines one uses to recognize a glass or a knife. Even if eyesight is primary in both cases, the intermodal links activated in conjunction with sight by the task of recognizing a face and those required by the recognition of a knife are just not the same. A face speaks, so what comes to the fore in the intermodal process is a linkage between eyesight and hearing; whereas a knife is handled, and so the processing of different types of visual data will be linked to the module dealing with tactile sensation.

Different Types of Intermodality

The relation between different modules should not be envisaged solely as a mere linkage. There are cases, of course, where it is completely missing, as in children who seem never to have made the connection between touch and sight (or sight and movement). Such children can give the impression that each of their domains functions in splendid isolation from all the others. It can also happen that an intermodal connection is made but in an ineffective way, because the eyesight is unable to play its proper organizing part. In the execution of a task that requires precision, it is often essential for the hand to be controlled by what can be gleaned about the situation from the eye. In the process, anything that the hand itself may be perceiving, either about its own movement or about the world around it, must also be attended to. Most importantly, such data still have to be organized in accordance with what the eye is registering. The quality of any intermodality depends on this leading role of the eyesight, and it is often this role that breaks down in the link between sight and touch or sight and movement.

Flexibility

At birth, every human being has a reflex for walking. If we simplify a little for the purposes of this discussion, this reflex can be considered as a network of predefined modular know-how. A few days after birth, the reflex is lost, and children then need to spend more than twelve months reacquiring the skill of walking. Can nature be out of joint? Is there a difference between reflex walking and acquired walking? Different studies that have been done show there are fundamental differences between the two ways of locomotion. The main difference is that reflex walking is a fixed program, made up of a sequence of stages that must be followed and that cannot be varied in any way (it is impossible to reach stage N without first going through stage N-1), whereas, in acquired walking, any of the stages can serve as the starting point for an original sequence. This enables humans, at any moment, to adapt their way of walking to the route to be taken, by choosing among the various versions of a particular stage according to need and in relation to the situation in which it tends to be utilized. This makes each stage into a kind of independent object. Cognitive evolution can actually be seen in a similar way. If, for example, intermodal links were fixed once for all, an object would be recognized only by one of its profiles and in a fixed context. But we must be able to recognize a thing under all circumstances, and recognition of it must also give us access to all the different knowledge we have acquired about it. Flexibility of intermodal connection is essential to the proper functioning of the modularity/intermodality combination. It appears that the key effect of cognitive maturation is to make for greater flexibility. What comes with age is greater scope for variability in the conditions of identification of an object, as well as the possibility of recognizing objects that are decontextualized from their usual setting and seen from any side or in unexpected situations. Once the object is recognized, age also gives better access to the whole set of data associated with it. Cognitive maturation leads to more flexible and more dependable intermodality. As a result, it is the demands of the object of perception that will determine intermodal links. This explains why visual recognition of a face does not happen in the same way as visual recognition of a knife or a corkscrew.

The Contribution of Developmental Psychology

So much for the account given in cognitive psychology of the reflex element in perception and action. It may be thought, however, that the most
important organizing of human activity takes place when the reflex mechanism is stalled and it becomes necessary to proceed to a more elaborate
strategy. Such a change often occurs after a brief depression, followed by
conscious thought that makes an unformed project into an explicit undertaking that can then be sustained and developed, even though it may not
be immediately attained. An intentional strategy of this sort cannot emerge
and supplant reflex chain reactions unless two conditions are met: subjects should have the ability to ignore part of what they perceive or "know,"
and they must also be able to focus attention on two things at once, for
instance, what they want (their purpose) and what they see (the effects of
their attempted actions).

Inhibition

Two fundamental indicators of cognitive maturation can be seen in the
ability to inhibit, avoid, or ignore either a reflex reaction or a particularly
attractive perception. This is what enables one to organize what one per-
ceives in terms of what one wants to do with it, rather than in terms of
the data inherent in whatever one discovers and finds intriguing.

As long ago as 1984, an article by David Premack gave a masterly account of the limits of animal behavior in this domain (Premack 1984).
He observed that a chimpanzee could spontaneously match half an apple
with half an apple and had little difficulty in matching a complete apple,
pear, or banana with the corresponding symbols. When the experimenter
complicated the animal's task by painting all of the fruit in a neutral color,
such as gray, the animal still performed well. When the fruit was painted
bright blue, things started to go wrong. And when the different fruits were
painted in bright but different colors (the banana blue, the apple indigo,
the pear red), the chimpanzee's performance "fell to chance" (Premack
1984, p. 185). The ape's surprise at the color of the painted fruit prevented it from inhibiting that dimension of the object and focusing on
shape recognition, which was the dimension that would have enabled it
to make the correct matches. It could not ignore a strange color; when
one particular dimension of a perceptible reality cannot be overlooked,

what results is a measure of fixity in the processes of intermodality. In order to change one's point of view on an object of perception, to ignore the color of it, even though it may be surprising, and focus on the shape of it, even though it may be ordinary (shape being the feature chosen as the basis of categorization), one must possess what Piaget called *décentrement*, the faculty of thinking beyond the self, which is what gives the ability to change one's point of view on an object.

The Ability to Manage Two Things at Once

Any subject who undertakes any intentional task is constrained to divide his or her attention. A baby, to take but one example, who is trying to reach a ball hanging above her cradle has her eyes fixed on it while with both hands she makes snatching movements that are at first clumsy and uncoordinated. The more she tries, the more her attempts become focused and organized, gradually leading to success. Unlike the reflex action, which gives a matching response without either trial or error, an intentional action requires a project, against which the successive attempts to carry it out will be assessed and rectified. This project must be sustained, but it must also be amended in the light of the lessons to be drawn from the unsuccessful attempts. Keeping the mind on what one wants and on the results of one's efforts to achieve what one wants is an essential aptitude. Many cognitive or symbolic processes demand the ability to attend to two things at once. Pointing is one of these processes: anyone pointing, at least anyone who wants to be sure of being understood, must keep two things in mind, the thing shown and the person to whom it is being shown. If one is incapable of managing two simultaneous centers of attention, one may well be incompetent at pointing.

Signs and Their Two Conditions

Those, then, are the few cognitive principles that I wanted to recapitulate before showing the effect they have on the very foundation of any sign.

All exchange relies on signs. A sign is a means of having somebody else feel and think the same as oneself. By virtue of being private experiences, however, thinking and feeling cannot be directly conveyed to another person. A detour is required, and it can be negotiated only under two conditions. First, one must establish a link between an inner feeling (a sensation) and an outer event that can constitute its visible side (the signifier). Then one must hold the belief that this link between the inner feeling and its visible side means for the other person what it means for you. Cognitive psychology suggests that both of these conditions derive from a particular type of innate intermodality.

Two Nipples

The link between the inner feeling and its visible side is strikingly illustrated by an experimentally established fact about babies (Mehler & Dupoux 1990). The test required a baby two weeks old to be offered two opaque feeding bottles, one with a rough nipple, the other with a smooth nipple. The bottle with the smooth nipple was empty; the one with the rough nipple contained milk. To begin with, the baby's eyes were covered, so that the nipples were invisible. It was only by mouth, through sucking, that the baby could tell that the bottle with the rough nipple was the full one. The second stage of the experiment consisted of letting the baby see the two bottles. Though the contents were invisible, it was observed that the baby's head immediately turned toward the bottle with the rough nipple. Since hitherto she had only felt it by mouth without seeing it, it must be supposed that the baby is equipped with a means of converting the perception of a feeling of roughness into a visual version of the same information. This must be what enables it to remember, on seeing the bottle with the rough nipple, that it is full of milk. Some cognitive psychologists take the view that this tells us something about the way our recognition of objects in the outside world functions. To me, it shows one of the ways in which signs are established: the rough nipple can be shown to someone else's eyes as a sign of sensations inside the mouth. Through this association, one contrives to signify to others a feeling they are not experiencing. Something that is internal, unrepresentable, and incommunicable in itself becomes associated with an external perception that plays the part of a signifier and makes the feeling accessible to others. A second condition, however, must be added: to make a sign, I must be able to think that the connection I make between signifier and signified has the same meaning for the person to whom I am addressing it. I propose now to look more closely at that second condition.

The Peanut and Babies Who Stick Out Their Tongues

A second experiment, recently done with monkeys but already familiar through studies of human babies, suggests that my second condition for the establishing of signs is also met (Fogassi et al. 1998; Rizzolatti et al. 1999). In the test, a monkey with electrodes wired to its head was offered a bowl containing glass marbles and a few peanuts, which the animal carefully extracted using its index finger and thumb. When it made this movement, a particular area of its brain, the one where the "mirror neurons" are, gave evidence of activity. In a second stage of the experiment, the monkey was shown one of the experimenters doing what it had done, finding a peanut among a bowl of marbles and taking it out, at which the monkey's neuronal activity followed the very same paths that it had taken while the monkey was taking the peanuts. In passing, a far from negligible point is that, if one replaces the peanut with something of less interest for the animal, a toy soldier, for instance, no evidence of neurological activity is recorded. The object manipulated must be one invested with meaning for the monkey. This means that, when the monkey seizes something of interest to it and when it sees someone else doing the same thing, it is the same areas of the brain that are activated. In other words, the sight of the experimenter taking the peanuts "evokes neuronally" for the monkey the potentiality for the action of seizing, if not an anticipatory experiencing of the sensation provided by the action. This, though a ground-breaking discovery in the field of monkeys, was not news in the field of babies. It was already known that, if you stick out your tongue at any baby that has the spontaneous ability to stick out its tongue, you can have a turn-taking exchange with it. The sight of the adult sticking out his or her tongue activates in the baby the representation of the action or the anticipation of the proprioceptive sensation of the action. This activation makes for tension, which the baby discharges by the effective reproduction of the movement of sticking out its own tongue. This turn-taking indicates a connection between perception and sensation. Here, though, unlike the experiment with the nipples, the connection is not between two different explorations of a single object in the world of inert things. No, this connection is one between a sensation linked to the proprioception of a movement made by the subject and the sight of the same movement made by someone else. This is one of the foundations of the imitative alternating behaviors that are among the earliest to be observed in very young children. It is also what guarantees to the child that a sign has the same meaning for others as for oneself.

In both experiments, the one with the nipples and the one with sticking out tongues, intermodality plays an essential part. In the first one, it guarantees the connection between a visible object (a signifier) and an invisible sensation (a signified). In the other one, it guarantees to any subject who makes the connection via a sign that this connection means for others what it means for the subject.

The organization of signs seems, therefore, to derive from two connections between sensation and visual perception that are radically different from each other. One of them comes about between visual perception and tactile exploration of an object; the other comes from the sight of an action done by someone else and the feeling of the same action done by oneself. Such innate linkages are clearly bound to be considerably developed in play between mother and child. Any mother who takes the trouble to stick out her tongue at her baby will be markedly enhancing the child's intermodal abilities.

Bundles of Thought

My intention here is to show how the construction of the bundles of thought that underlie exchange can be adversely affected by a disorder of intermodality and of the ability to think beyond the self. It is conceivable that a cognitive disorder, whether of eyesight, motor skills, or the link between them, may be the source of certain types of difficulty encountered by children in the construction of notions preparatory to any putting into words. When a child does not have the possibility of converting, associating, and modulating his different modes of knowledge of an object, when his image of it, his tactile impression, the smell of it, the sounds it makes, its ways of occupying space do not spontaneously come together, when he has access to such data only separately, then his ways of thinking and speaking will become complex, strange, and invariable. What is affected is presumably not his words but rather his construction of the notions that precede his words. I have just mentioned the lack of interconnectedness between data of diverse nature that derive from a single object. But sometimes the cause lies in a difficulty with imagining the actions that might go with a given situation. This can translate, for example, into an inability to conceive of the way to handle an object properly, which may affect the most habitual sort of action, such as how to lift a glass to one's lips, or actions that are less bound by circumstance, such as thinking up a set of actions for a puppet in an invented sketch: if a glass or a puppet bring nothing to mind, any story that can develop out of them quickly becomes disjointed or very thin.

From Bundles of Thought to Categories

A prerequisite for the construction of the notions that serve as the basis of lexical words is the existence of lexico-referential categories. However, these categories are of a rather peculiar sort. This can be seen instantly in the fact, for example, that a sparrow, a penguin, an ostrich, and a cock are all birds. In fact, as Wittgenstein and then Eleanor Rosch pointed out long ago, a category does not entail bringing together an assemblage of identical individuals or even of individual specimens all of which share one or more properties (Wittgenstein 1953; Rosch 1977). It may be the case, of course, that pairs of individuals of similar type do share some properties, but no property is, strictly speaking, shared by all individuals of the set. To construct types, it has to be possible to define the properties that justify putting the sparrow and the cock together (flying and pecking up seeds, for instance), then to leave aside those two features and establish another link between, say, the penguin and the cock. Without this, the penguin cannot be thought of as a bird. It is clear that such juggling with properties, first giving pride of place to one of the properties of an object, then letting it recede so as to focus on another one, depends on the cognitive ability to ignore whichever features of an object one has decided are not relevant. This requires constant changes of point of view and the ability to bring about what Piaget calls *décentrement*, thinking beyond the self.

Decontextualization

This skill of seeing things from points of view different from one's own is one of the most surprising that any child can learn; it is what makes children capable of recognizing the same object in radically dissimilar contexts. One may well be struck by the fact that, by the age of eighteen months, the human infant is able to say *de l'eau* (= "[some] water") when he wants to be given some in a glass, when a drop of rain falls on his nose and he dislikes the feeling of wet, when he is in his bath and wants some more warm water added, or when he discovers the sea on arriving for the first time at a beach. All these contexts are profoundly different from one another, a fact that does not seem to be a problem. Against that, we know that autistic children have the acutest difficulty in using words outside the confines of the immediate situation in which they first heard them. Leo Kanner, in one of his ground-breaking cases, tells the story of a child to whom the word "yes" never meant anything except a way of asking to be sat up on someone's shoulders, because this was the context in which he had used the word for the first time. The way in which a child's referential vocabulary becomes established makes it possible to devise hypotheses about this gradual growth of indifference to context. If we take the standard onomatopoeia *ouah* (= "woof"), meaning a dog, we can see three rough stages. To begin with, the word is reserved exclusively for a particular animal in a particular situation (the family's dog, for instance). Then it gets applied not just to all dogs but to cats or horses encountered in books or on outings. Finally, the word comes to be used only in connection with the appropriate referents and is reserved for dogs. This development could lend itself to different explanations. The one it suggests to me is that, at first, what makes it possible to recall representations of objects is the memory of the events, the contexts, and the particular circumstances of our encounter with them. In other words, at the beginning, what induces the use of words in a child (with the memory of the thing corresponding to the words) is the situation in which he happens to be: it reminds him of another situation with which the object is associated. At this stage, the process of recall brings back to mind not the object's own properties but only the situation and the scenario in which it figured. In the next stage, the properties of the object come into play. The dominant memory system is no longer the one that retains the events experienced by a subject but the one that is grounded in the properties of things. Semantic memory becomes more important than memory related to events. This is what frees the recall of an object from the context from which it was originally inseparable. Soon a property will recall all the objects that have it, which can lead to comparisons that strike us as strange, like the one where the child sees a horse and says *ouaoua* (= "woof woof"). This does not mean that the child actually thinks the horse is a dog. All he is doing is making a link between the present horse and the memory of the dog. The look of the horse brings the dog to mind because a horse, like a dog, is a quadruped that makes a particular sound. More time will be required for the word to be reserved for the objects that really correspond to it.

The cognitive point of view helps to clarify some aspects of disorders relating to the use of signs. It can also serve to identify disorders in lexical categories. What it does not do is explain why certain children do not speak, there being obviously no simple explanation for that. Nevertheless, one can always formulate hypotheses, which is what the following chapter is about.

14

Why Do Some Children Not Communicate?

The way we speak to these children, or, to be more accurate, our way of making sense a posteriori of our dealings with them, depends on whatever hypotheses we have formulated about the possible sources of their disorder. This is especially pertinent when one goes from speech disorders to the area of childhood psychosis and autism, where the so-called disorder of communication becomes severe.

By and large, descriptions of communication disorders have been relatively consensual: points of view may differ, but the focus is on the same symptoms. It is on the meaning to be attached to the symptoms that hypotheses diverge. There is a divide between specialists who look to psychoanalysis for explanations and those who look to cognition; between these two different ways of defining the problem, there are predictably fierce differences of opinion. The cognitive scientists speak of deficiencies or malfunctions in the neurological mechanism. They take the view that these children lack what is necessary to the making of appropriate contacts and social interactions. The psychoanalysts speak of defense. They take the view that, to children who are autistic or psychotic, contact with another person is so agitating that they have to take refuge in delirium or withdrawal. From this divide there follows a basic difference in the treatments proposed. For the cognitive scientist, what is required is re-education and remediation; for the psychoanalyst, what is required is interpretation and making sense. This makes for two positions that are diametrically irreconcilable. To my way of thinking, however, as I said in connection with dysphasia, neither of them seems tenable. What is indisputable is that, in the case of children with severely disturbed communication, there is "something wrong with" the functioning of the instrument and that the "something" that is "wrong with" it is bound to be one of the sources of the disorder in the psychic processes. In communication, any child who cannot interpret the signs being addressed to him is constantly being thrust into the unforeseeable. This causes the terror and extreme agitation to which withdrawal is a response. To be always in the presence of somebody who is making signs that one cannot identify, that one cannot link to a representation linking in turn with something known, is to be constantly in the presence of the unthinkable. Anyone who has ever set foot in a foreign country and felt lost amid an unknown language and customs has had a similar disconcerting experience. Comprehension being at best fragmentary, one eventually withdraws into oneself, converting an instrumental disorder into self-defense, much as a deaf person copes with a malfunctioning hearing aid by switching it off, preferring total silence to partial understanding. The defect in the equipment lies at the origin of agitation or withdrawal. But it is the reinforcement of the defect itself that is the first defense chosen by the subject. It would take a measure of masochism to put up with the agitation caused by not properly understanding messages addressed to oneself. So, when understanding breaks down, one can have a quieter life if one just drops out.

The Different Positions

Going back to the different theoretical positions, one can say that anyone who attempts to define the meaning and import of disorders of nonverbal and prelinguistic communication has a choice between cognitive psychology and psychoanalysis. If one favors the cognitive approach, one will conclude that the disorder of communication derives from a difficulty with imagining the mind of someone else. This supposes that an autistic child who has not acquired a "theory of mind," who is thereby unable to conceive of how mental states can affect people's actions and give meaning to them, will be incapable of communicating or of relating socially in any satisfactory way.

Against that, there is the psychoanalytical approach, a basic tenet of which says in effect that a child with a communication disorder (who avoids contact and retreats into prostration or into rituals that keep everything at a distance) is a child who cannot work out how to be with other people, whether because he is in thrall to their influence upon him or because he cannot contrive to think of himself as separate. Since any exchange presupposes a relatively stable degree of separateness between those who engage in it, no child with such psychic disorders can ever establish coherent communication.

A third order of explanation holds that the disorders of the autistic child are caused by "dismantling," the term used in psychoanalysis (Meltzer 1975) or by dissociation, the term used in cognitive science. Here, strangely enough, the two points of view intersect; it is at this intersection that I propose to add another point of view, in part of my own devising. This suggestion, which owes as much to cognitive science as it does to psycho-analysis, consists of stressing the fact that a child who lacks the ability to establish a proper relation between sensation and perception may have particular difficulty in constructing and interpreting any sign. Therein, I suggest, lies the dismantling (or the specific dissociation) in question.

A Possible Weakness in the "Theory of Mind" Theory

The account given of autistic syndromes by some theorists in cognitive science, for instance Uta Frith (Baron-Cohen et al. 1985), postulates an organic deficit that deprives the child of the reflexes essential to the in-terpretation of signs as expressed by faces, particularly in the register of feelings and the use of the eyes.

According to this idea, the child's problem stems from an inability to read emotions or to gauge what someone else is looking at from the posi-tion of a person's head or the direction of the glance. Unable to assess the feelings of others or to discover what interests them, autistic children, it is said, have neither empathy nor any representation of someone else's representation. Nor do they have the idea of showing anyone else what they themselves find interesting. This would explain why they do not point, since pointing presupposes the belief that another person can share one's interests. The "aloneness" of the autistic child could thus be explained as deriving from a minor, selective neurological disorder. This hypothesis is supported by various observations, notably the fact that high-functioning children with autism do appear to have greater difficulty in matching photographs of faces according to their expressions (e.g., fear, pleasure, anger) or the direction of their eyes than according to other, more "ob-jective" criteria, such as their general shape. This theory, which I have just sketched in its broad lines, is open to several criticisms. First, to say that an autistic child has no representation of another person's mind is incompatible with what can be observed. It is common that when an autistic child wants something, he will take your hand and move it toward whatever it is that he is trying to get. A demonstration of this sort presupposes a representation of another's mind. It may be neither as disinterested nor as unambiguous as the same thing done by a normal child, but for all its impairment and awkwardness, it still exists. From a clinical point of view, it is this very awkwardness that has to be assessed. Second, an ability to read facial signs is undoubtedly a necessary condition for looking at whatever someone else is looking at, but it is certainly not a sufficient condition. In order to look at what someone else is looking at, one must want to do so. And yet to do so requires one of the most painful and complex efforts that a human soul is capable of. When somebody starts to look at something other than yourself, you are forgotten: to look at what the other person is looking at, you must accept that you are no longer of interest, that something (or someone) else is more interesting than you, and you must also take an interest in whatever is being looked at. A baby who can look at what his mother is looking at when she turns away from him is admittedly a baby who is able to read her face, but he is also a baby who is able to engage with what his mother engages with, even though it may be to his own disadvantage.

Third, the cognitive perspective also posits that a child who cannot interpret other people's eye movements will never be able to establish joint attention with anyone. However, there is nothing inevitable about this: being unable to decipher facial expressions is not an irremediable obstacle to the construction of joint attention. In a therapeutic setting, even with a child who cannot point at something of interest to him (and on condition that the child is not immured in total withdrawal), it is possible to organize a shared point of exchange. To cite one example among others, this is exactly what happens when the child is looking out the window at the darkness and one comments on the passing cars. If this is to lead to anything, there are of course several necessary conditions, the first of which is to have nothing to do with a theory that argues that this is impossible. Next, we must be prepared to take an interest in what interests the child, by meeting him on his own ground and not obliging him to meet us on ours. Also, we must sit or stand beside and not opposite him, so as to be looking in the same direction, and one must comment. Not that it follows from this that such a child will then point. Using a finger to point something out is a more complex operation, requiring

the ability to make someone who has no spontaneous interest in something share your focus on it. It is this second level that is inaccessible to
children with communication disorders. Occasionally, however, even
some of those who cannot manage to achieve it will accept someone who
tries to share their focus of attention. I stress that this happens only on
occasion, it being well known that most of the time one can look at what
the child is looking at without the slightest outcome of any sort. That
very fact, by the way, also suggests that the establishment of joint attention depends on more conditions than the straightforward neurological
aptitude of reading others' intentions from their facial expressions.

The Evolution of the "Theory of Mind" Theory

Since its early days, the "theory of mind" theory has evolved, and today
there are several differentiated hypotheses that distinguish between various degrees of complexity. Children differ: some of them do credit another person with a representation of the present situation, and possibly
with feelings, intentions, and beliefs, as well. Importantly, however, tests
designed for the purpose of examining these new hypotheses have produced some disturbing findings. The first is that, unlike what can be observed in other cases of limited neuropsychological deficits (certain
neurological disorders of eyesight, for example), the performances of
autistic subjects are extremely variable. They are affected by the context and the moment at which the child performs. A stranger thing is
that their performances in the tests appear to be better than those in
ordinary life: a child who finds it difficult to anticipate someone else's
mental reactions in their daily dealings will manage it better, relatively
speaking, under laboratory conditions. This variability suggests that the
disorder in childrens' theory of mind as observed in autism might be
the result not so much of a defect in the neurological circuitry (if that
were the case, there would be no variation in the disorder) as of a defect in the activation of the circuits, and that might be produced by
malfunctioning secretions of brain hormones. The neurotransmitters
might function intermittently. The fact that performances under ordinary conditions differ from those in the laboratory might indicate that
the child's central difficulty concerns the selecting of indicators enabling
choices of behavior appropriate to given situations. For it is the case that,
in experimental situations, the indicators that lead to a choice of strategy

are more salient, more stable, and more controlled than those in ordinary situations. Or a further reason for the disparity could be that there is a particular memory difficulty. With events or actions that have just happened, there are children who appear to have a problem with instantaneous recall, which prevents them from reproducing such an event or action or from using it as the starting point for behavior of their own. They seem to need an initial moment's forgetting before they can exploit what their memory has recorded; if this is the case, it is quite understandable that such an enforced suspension of memory should provoke a disconnection that compromises interaction of any sort, for in the sequential exchanges of everyday life every event has to immediately condition any response to it.

Autism and Frontal Disorders

Some accounts of patients with frontal syndromes, due either to hormonal malfunctions or neurological impairment, can suggest striking analogies with the difficulties experienced by autistic children. It is an intriguing parallel that certainly bears thinking about (Damasio and Maurer 1978; Adrien et al. 1993; Mazeau 1997).

Put simply, frontal disorders are of three kinds: disorders of mood and emotion; difficulties in initiating intentional acts (lack of initiative); and attention disorders.

Descriptions of the first kind stress the patients' taciturnity or its opposite, an excessive ebullience or even lewdness in speech. They bring to mind autistic children who are either severely withdrawn or so agitated that they can calm themselves down only by resorting to their stereotypies or to masturbatory practices. Both groups are marked by excessive moods that are insensitive to accepted norms of social behavior. Also attributable to this mood disorder are the voice, either toneless or overmodulated, that is often found in both of these pathologies. This disorder could even explain the trouble that both sorts of patients experience in reading other people's emotions and taking account of these in their interactions with them.

Lack of initiative, the second set of difficulties, shows in the fact that adults with frontal disorders are frequently as incapable as any autistic child of undertaking intentional action, which is replaced by inertness or the unremitting repetition of stereotyped acts. Repetition is the concomitant of an inability to develop intentional activity, though perhaps it could be argued that the nub of the problem lies in the lack of initial impetus. When a "frontal" patient or an autistic child is at a loss for an appropriate action, sometimes a hint or a helping hand from someone else, though minimal and unbiased, may be enough to get the subject to start an action or carry it through. What can be very striking in such situations is that the hint or helping hand is in no way an instruction about which action to take. This finding underlies various rather curious techniques in which the therapist supports the child's hand by way of helping her to write or type on a keyboard. In such sessions, it may well be asked whether the therapist is not actually prompting the text produced by the patient. There are cases, however, where this is certainly not true and the therapist does no more than give an impetus, without feature or particular direction, that helps the child carry out an act.

The third of these difficulties, attention disorder, manifests itself in many dissimilar forms. Two different types of attention should be defined: there is attentiveness, the alertness of the senses, a heightened readiness to perceive, unfocused on any objective; and there is attention proper, aimed at a goal to be attained. The latter is the mode of attention most commonly disordered. It demands a set of different things: that a subject be able to think of what he wants and of what he is doing to achieve what he wants, while adapting his strategies as he goes along. In addition, he must be capable of inhibiting any perception unrelated to his aim and any inappropriate action, such as a reflex or an obsolete strategy. To put it another way, the subject must know what he wants and understand what he sees, while at the same time managing to keep things in perspective, to be both focused and flexible. Also, given that actions developing over time require one to see different aspects of situations, he must have the ability to see things from a perspective other than one's own. What all this amounts to is the broad repertory of skills required by the planning and carrying out of a complex motor sequence.

The Nonindividuation Hypothesis

I propose now to revert to the range of problems that standard psychoanalysis sees as explaining the difficulties of autistic children. Here, the central idea is that, to communicate, any subject has to accept the feeling of being separate from the object of his love. Any child in whom this process of individuation has not occurred has recourse to two avoidance strategies. The first of these is withdrawal, whereby he shuts himself off in total solitude, away from any relation with others; the second consists of seeing himself in a state of constant fusion with others. With a child in that state, no exchange is possible, since any speech or action addressed to somebody else must presuppose that the person speaking or acting accepts that there is a distance between them. If this initial distance does not exist, nothing can happen. This is the reasoning most commonly put forward by way of explanation of the lack of speech and communication in children suffering from disorders of a psychotic or autistic kind.

This makes for a convincing description. However, to my mind, it jumps rather too quickly to the conclusion that a child who never addresses anyone else does not know she is separate from anyone else. I find it difficult to accept that the experience of her senses (sight, hearing, smell, touch) should be utterly incapable of contradicting the illusion of a seamless continuity between her and the person she declines to address. I am aware that there are perceptions that remain inoperative because they are not invested with interest by the child. Nonetheless, rather than read into this the idea that the child lives in total ignorance of her separation from others, it appears to me more to the point to assume that such a child is actually refusing to acknowledge this severance between herself and others, despite the fact that each of her senses is a source of possible contradiction of her refusal. In my view, such an unspeaking child is only too aware of the distance that separates her from others. She knows it, but she is reluctant to recognize it, whether through speech or exchange. The reason she does not communicate is not that she senses no distinction between herself and others but rather that she believes communicating would force her to abandon her illusion of seamless continuity between her and others. Speaking would be tantamount to abandoning the illusion; until something can change in that, she prefers only self-addressed speech or else silence. This way of redefining the problem has immediate therapeutic consequences: a child who does not communicate can be brought to speak on condition that the exchange does not force her to acknowledge her separation from others. She can be brought to see the point of dialogue and engage in it via a variable use of speech situations that maintain a degree of relative fusion between her and others. The extent of the psychic differentiation implicit in communication is, in fact, flexible enough to lend itself to modulation. This idea lies at the heart of how I approach such children.

Dismantling and Dissociation

The lack of individuation is not the only theory on autism developed by psychoanalysts. Donald Meltzer has a different one, which explains the disorders observed in autistic behavior as a "dismantling" of the faculties as a whole. According to Meltzer, because there is insufficient connection between information received from different sources and insufficient connection with affect, the child becomes engrossed in the pleasures afforded by isolated sensations that come to his body from contact with outer reality. In so doing, he prevents any representation from forming. Meltzer sees this as a defense set up against being overwhelmed and disorganized by the presence of another person. Curiously enough, cognitive science has borrowed unawares several hypotheses that are consistent with this idea, though the name given to the process is not "dismantling" but "dissociation." Dissociation affects the child at various points, impairing either the links between the different modules of perception or the way in which variability of point of view can facilitate understanding of the world. For most people, processing any state of reality entails the necessity to see it both as a whole and as a set of separate elements, while weighing each of these perspectives against the other. What is very noticeable in autistic children is, of course, that they make a radical dissociation between these two ways of experiencing external reality (Mottron et al. 1999).

My own preferred position coincides with the general hypothesis of dismantling. One of the sources of autistic children's inability to communicate lies in their radical dissociation between sensation and perception; connection between these two faculties is essential to the establishment of signs and the ability to communicate.

The Essential Connection between Sensation and Perception

Communicating is an attempt to share with someone a fact, a sensation, an affect, a purpose, a state of feeling, or an idea that lies nowhere but in one's own head or heart. It is self-evident that one cannot make what lives inside one's body directly visible to other people. One can ask them to pay attention to a sound or to some visible event; but one can give no direct access to any feeling or thought that one harbors. Hence, one falls back on the use of outside objects, which one offers to others as a signifier betokening that inward reality. Communicating is designating a directly audible, palpable, or visible object of perception in the expectation that for someone else it will "stand for" the inner state that one wishes to convey. A straightforward example is the inner state known as sadness, which one can contrive to communicate only by a show of something (like tears, cries, or a facial expression of distress) that another person, through sight, touch, or hearing, can associate with one's state. As I have said, it is this association between sensation and perception that profoundly disturbed children lack. In maintaining this, I am doing no more than making inferences from propositions that are relatively well established. It is an assumption that coincides with the view, current in cognitive psychology, that stresses the breakdown of intermodality in some children with severe problems of communication. It is also consistent with the psychoanalytical idea of "dismantling." Striking examples of it can be seen in the behavior of certain patients who are able to manipulate objects while looking at something completely different. When an autistic child can spin a wine glass with his finger and vaguely inspect the ceiling at the same time (I have seen it done), it must mean that each of his sensory processes can function separately from the others. This tendency to dissociation prevents any linkage being made between sensation and perception. And the consequence is that the construction of signs is not feasible.

I would go farther: I do not believe it is only the conveying of thought and inner states that is affected by dissociation between sensation and perception. I also suspect that deprivation of this linkage makes it impossible for any subject to have a self-representation of anything he or she may feel. And anyone who wishes to remember his or her own sensation, while being incapable of having a representation of it, is doomed to repeat it ad infinitum.

Here, too, what I am proposing is consonant with positions already agreed upon. There is a strain of psychoanalytical thinking that sees the basis of all our affects and our representations (that is, possibly the whole substance of any representational activity) as being composed of innermost states of feeling or bodily sensations. There is a diversity of these: coenesthetic and kinesthetic, and those relating to posture, balance, and touch. These are what disturbs the body's stable state and makes the psyche think. But they are also what is transformed during the very process of representation. This point of view informs the work of Didier Anzieu (Anzieu 1984, 1987, 1995).

The Status of Sensations

As is well known, standard Freudian thinking posits the existence of a "primary" process, which precedes not just any activity that translates thought into words but also the transition to preconscious thought, and it is here that fantasies linked to the representations of things can be created. But even that primary activity is not the most basic ground of consciousness. According to Anzieu, what underlies all psychic functioning is an accumulation of innermost states of feeling and bodily sensations, or "formal signifiers," a term he borrows from Guy Rosolato (Rosolato 1984), which precedes any activity of the primary process. This corresponds to the area for which Piera Castoriadis-Aulagnier has proposed the term *l'originaire* (= "the originary [area]") (Castoriadis-Aulagnier 1975). These innermost sensations, lying at the heart of all representation, emanate from within the body, in which their presence is ineradicable, corresponding to postural changes of the type "open/closed," "collapse," "explode," "attached/unattached," or "strained." These are fragmentary, scattered, and shapeless impressions, devoid of real contours or content, hardly comparable to one another, akin to those from muscular tension, from leaning against something, or a throb, proprioceptions of acts or movement, events impossible to relate to any organized form, and never anything approaching perceptions traceable to stable external objects.

From Sensation to Representation

Bodily sensations are strong disturbances, though unrepresentable as such. If any representation of them is to be achieved, it has to be made from material that is radically different from what they are made of. Recourse must be had to visual and auditory perception, the source of which is external. This is actually what one does when trying to give form to an inner sensation. A sensation of falling or losing balance translates in the mind as a vertical landscape rolling past or a glimpse of someone falling over. In both cases, the representation content is visual. Were it not for this resort to perception whose source is outside the self, what is felt within the body, the impression of something tightening, slipping, or dropping away, remains unrepresentable. Inner sensation can come to representation only through perception contents that are visual or auditory. These function as a sign and a representation for inner sensation. Every subject is obliged to associate his or her inner sensations with perceptible variations from the outside world. Otherwise, no subject can bring them to representation; in order to remember them, the subject can do nothing other than repeat them.

The Development of the Link between Sensation and Perception

The connection between sensation and perception is in part innate, a point that has been stressed by cognitive scientists and demonstrated in the experiments with the rough nipple and the monkey and the peanut. But this connection becomes properly organized only through the very early interactions between mother and child. It is these interactions that foster the growth and solidity of associations between proprioceptive contents of a sensation kind and perceptive contents received from the remoter functioning of the different senses. In this, the music and materiality of the mother's speech constitute an essential link, ensuring that representation can eventually be organized with stability and flexibility into a construction that is solid but alterable. During these early interactions, the mother's voice comes between the infant's inner experience (its sensations) and all its various perceptions from the outside world, especially the visual ones.

Take the example of a baby being cuddled and sung to. The perception of the sound of the mother's song enables the baby to have a representation of its sensations. To feel them again, he can listen internally to his mother singing. This singing becomes the baby's first representation of being cradled in her arms and sung to. A mother can, of course, do this in a great many different situations; in each of these, the baby will see and experience something different. The mother's voice not only helps to stabilize the baby's inner experience of its sensations; it also promotes a multiplicity of relations among all the diverse things that the baby discovers on each occasion. The speaking voice of the mother is thus in a pivotal position, not just stabilizing the baby's representation of its own inner experiences but also mediating a relation between these and a great variety of visual perceptions. This is how it becomes the signified of a whole range of images that correspond to the single circumstance of being cradled and sung the same song in different situations. So the voice is the perceptible matter most easily associated with the inner sensation that it helps to stabilize. But it also represents an indefinite number of potential visual situations, all different from one another and any one of which can work as a sort of metaphor for the lullaby. With the child in danger of autism, however, the sound of the mother's voice does not occupy that strategic place. In those circumstances, all there is is a relation that is direct, static, and unalterable between an inner experience and an outer image. This way of seeing the problem leads us to understand that, when an autistic child manages, despite his difficulties, to organize an association, it always remains static, and the child finds it forever impossible to associate an object (or a sign) with different contexts or meanings. As a result, if any new association is to be possible, the previous one has to be abolished.

Stereotypy as a Failed Attempt at Self-Cure

To be thought about, represented, and spoken of, an inner state must first be linked to something seen or heard, whose source is sensed as being outside the body. When sensations, of which the body is the host, have no connection with what is outside the body, they are unrepresentable and become threatening. This elementary statement of fact (I cannot talk about what I feel in my body unless I relate this to changes that happen outside it and are perceptible to other people) seems to me to cast a particularly revealing light on some of the clinical data on autism. A hypothesis that has often been advanced is that autistic children find within themselves bodily sensations that are unrepresentable. If this is the case, it may be because the ordinary innate link between experience of such sensations and visual and auditory perceptions has not been established, just as there has been a breakdown in the other natural link (found in babies who can imitate an adult sticking out his tongue) between seeing someone do something and doing it oneself. The whole system of representations is upset by this. Nothing is foreseeable, for one thing; for another, whatever does happen in the child's vicinity is an encroachment into his own space. The unpredictability of things makes him also unpredictable, which disturbs the early relation with the mother. In the most serious cases, the mother's speech cannot even establish the intermodal links that were absent in the first place.

Under such circumstances, falling back on stereotypy is the only way to set up limits and give some shape to inner sensations that are ungraspable in any other way. An autistic child who moves a hand in front of her eyes is presumably ridding herself of the tension that may be caused by the presence of somebody else. But it may also be an attempt to connect what she feels when she waves an arm in front of a lamp with the alternation between light and shade caused by her hand movement. Stereotypy is an effort to make a relation between the muscular sensation felt in the moving wrist and the impressions of light resulting from the movement of her hand. Every stereotypy may be considered as a way of relating a visual or auditory perception with a kinesthetic sensation (balance or tactile). This is the basic meaning of repetitions such as swaying to and fro, opening and closing things, pulling them and letting go, taking and leaving them. The purpose of the action is to give some figurable form to the shapeless inner sensations of the subject by giving them the focus of a perception. Similarly, a child who keeps picking up a piece of folded cardboard from a table top and dropping it again is presumably trying to stabilize his agitation. However, he is also presumably trying to make a connection between the sensation he gets from opening and closing his hand and his visual perception of the piece of cardboard dropping, as well as the sound it makes on the table. Since the contact between his perceptions (the sight of it falling, the sound it makes) and the sensation of opening his hand is momentary, he is bound to keep on making it by repeating the action. Stereotypy is an attempt at mastering sensations that have become unrepresentable through their severance from the perceptible. If this link is not stabilized, if sensations cannot be durably associated with perception, then all sensation must forever remain in a limbo from which there is no access to representation or affect and where the only way of controlling it is to repeat it.

Conclusion

In the fourth part of this book, I have recapitulated some general hypotheses on the way communication and language become organized, and I have canvassed the relative causal importance of the neurological mechanism and the psychic process when either communication or language is disordered. Some of the children to whom I have referred are best seen as suffering from neurosis, and their language difficulties are massive. Others, above and beyond their language difficulties, also have a disorder in communication. It is this similarity with childhood psychosis that, in accordance with common Anglo-American practice, sometimes leads to their being classified as autistic. My own feeling is that, in both cases, the neurological mechanism is seriously implicated. That much is obvious, if there is a language disorder; in my view, it must also be true of disordered communication. In the latter case, the disorder takes effect at the stage where notions translatable as words are organized before being put into words. This has often been mentioned in discussion of pathologies that fall short of full-blown autism.

In all cases, it is of course important to recognize neurological deficiencies or distortions, while at the same time gauging and defining the psychic implications of them. This is exactly what I try to do in my therapeutic practice. My purpose is never to reeducate a child or bury him under a heap of interpretations, any more than it is to leave him to his own devices in the hope that he will just get better. One of my purposes is to play the part of someone to whom a sign fraught with affect is addressed, to acknowledge this for the person addressing it to me, and to show him or her that the meaning of it can be shared. This approach derives from ideas, from things observed and things read. These ideas are what I have tried to set forth in this book. They all focus on the fact that the ability to acquire language and communication is affected by heterogeneous factors that can be roughly seen as cohering around three different axes. The first of these, the cognitive axis, is related to how any speaker has constructed his experience of and interaction with the world. In the world, there are other human beings who very often mediate the domain of the inert and who serve as interlocutors in speech exchange. This is why attention must be paid to how the speaker relates to them. The second axis concerns the mechanics of speech, with its connections to the speech apparatus. This is the register that is missing in aphasic patients, the mechanism that makes it possible to put ideas and feelings into words and to understand the meaning of what is said. The third axis is the one that, as a psychoanalyst, I see as most important: symbolization. Every utterance, every communication, makes audible and visible the way any signifying subject relates his thinking (his representations) to the world of which he speaks and to the thinking he presupposes in whoever is listening to him. This definition by a subject of the relationship between his representations and the world, of the minds of others, and of his own mind is decisive. I describe it as symbolization to distinguish it from representation: representation is about contents; symbolization is about perspectives on contents. Any one of these three focuses may be beset by disturbances that will have an unavoidable effect on observable utterances. I have tried to indicate ways in which such disturbances may be made sense of, notably as concerns the link between sensation and perception. None of this should be taken to mean that I think I have understood everything. There are times, when one is working with children in difficulty, when one can feel rather low and the temptation to theorize can appear to be a good idea. Theory is a powerful antidepressant. It can, however, like any efficacious molecule, have side effects, such as skepticism or clannish adherence to one's school of thought. In this book, as a linguist and a psychoanalyst, I have tried to bring together some basic facts on symbolization as seen from the perspective afforded by the pathology of communication and language. It is almost a century since Ernst Cassirer drew up his classification of symbolic forms. Here, my aim has been to bring out the conditions under which such forms can prosper or may be inhibited. It can be difficult to know with any certainty whether one is faced with an instrumental disorder that is merely manifesting itself in the symbolic register or with a psychic disorder derived from an impairment in the processing of drives and representation. In many cases, these two disorders appear together: if one has constant trouble finding words, speaking may make for more anxiety than enjoyment, even when one is talking to oneself; and being forever unable to understand what others are saying can make for madness. A semblance of control over this can be the resort to ritual; the risk this entails is that it may lead to the sterility of repetitiveness.

In a way, my therapeutic endeavor is to avoid that outcome and to foster the unpredictable, as well as to indulge my own liking for a mode of creative passivity—which is why all my activity amounts to an extended comment on the meaning of the word "language" itself. This, at least, is where I concur with the *Glossaire* of Michel Leiris and the poetic definition he gives of the word: *Langage : engage au jeu par élan* (= "Language: urges to play by impulse").[1]

---

1. Translator's note: Michel Leiris's poetic punning is untranslatable, alas, in any way that preserves the puns or the poetry, which is all in semiphonetic anagram.

Glossary

abstract play: see page 96.

addressee: person toward whom communication is directed and who can have an important bearing on the quality of the sign produced by the addresser.

affect: affect expresses what we feel about what we think or experience. Unlike emotions, affect has mental, conative, or representational associations. Like emotions, however, affects can be communicated via gesture or facial expressions. Some children with a communication disorder find it difficult to express them.

agent: term used in semantics for the person or thing that does an action, for example, the subject "Jean" in the sentence "Jean eats an apple" or "train" in the passive statement "Jean was run over by a train."

anatomopathology: study of the human anatomy (particularly the brain) and of the relations between a disorder (a pathology) and its anatomical localization in the brain.

animal behavior: behaviors studied are usually those of primates, especially their capacities for abstraction, symbolization, and socialization. Some studies try to identify animal origins for certain specifically human behaviors, for example, can monkeys draw the attention of other monkeys to things by pointing at them?

animate/inanimate: see page 100.

anthropomorphized play: see page 96.

aphasiological disorder: disorder akin to aphasia in adults, though not necessarily accompanied by any organic lesion.

apraxia: inability to perform purposeful movements, unrelated to paralysis.

approximation: cognitive process of definition of an object by association with a category to which it is recognized as not belonging but to which it is close.

aspect: see page 179.

Asperger's syndrome: autistic spectrum disorder in children who speak and are in general gifted but whose relations with others are markedly awkward. These children are often gifted in some areas, such as languages, yet show great difficulty in others, such as math. Behavioral symptoms include a difficulty with eye contact when speaking to an addressee and certain peculiarities of language (misuse of pronouns, odd intonations). Such children can engage in exchange with others and be tolerably well integrated socially.

attention disorder: see page 219.

attunement: term used by Daniel Stern for the way a mother "instinctively" regulates her affects and rhythms in accordance with those of her child.

audimutism: more or less equivalent to profound dysphasia, possibly linked to a massive disorder in language reception.

autism: pathological relational and communication disorder, marked by aloneness; avoidance of eye contact; ritual behaviors and dislike of change; stereotypy (e.g., spinning around, hand-flapping); language disorder, ranging from total absence of language to echolalia, misuse of pronouns ("you" instead of "I"), odd intonations; phobias associated with eating or sounds; self-damage.

automatic speech: see page 52.

autonomy of sound and movement: see page 86.

bodily sensations: coenesthetic and kinesthetic, and those relating to posture, balance, and touch. They are what disturb the body's stable state and make us think. But they are also what will be transformed during the process of representation. See especially the work of Didier Anzieu.

Broca's aphasia: adult aphasia characterized by a degree of difficulty in producing articulate speech. Differs from Wernicke's aphasia (neurological inability to identify the sounds of language).

categorization: cognitive process in which an object is compared to a set of objects sharing a common property with it, enabling the formation of analogies and differences (A is like B on this point but unlike B on that one). Children often follow this mode of investigation, learning to organize their world and to see themselves in relation to it. Basic resemblances enable the recognition of differences. The process works only if a child has the capacity for *décentrement* (see definition).

child aphasia: "aphasia," meaning loss of language already acquired, is not normally used for children. However, it may be used in referring to a young child who has lost acquired language, for instance as a result of an accident.

child psychoanalysis: differs from adult psychoanalysis in that it works mainly through the use of play and drawing. Begun by Freud, greatly developed by Melanie Klein, Anna Freud, and Donald Winnicott.

child psychosis: category used in the French nosographical tradition differently from in the English-speaking world. In French nosography it is defined by a loss of sense of reality, a propensity to fantasize, and sometimes incoherent utterances. The psychotic child retains the ability to represent the real world without the fragmentation of dissociation of perceptions. He or she can also maintain contact with others, though this may be idiosyncratic. These two factors distinguish this category of pathology from autism proper. Some nosographical definitions equate it with "pervasive developmental disorder" or "semantic-pragmatic syndrome." However, in pervasive developmental disorder, contrary to psychosis, there is no distortion of reality, the category being defined much more functionally.

cognitive dimension: one of the three dimensions in which a serious disturbance of a child's language may manifest itself, the other two being the aphasiological and the symbolic. Cognitive disorder refers to the child's neurological difficulties, for example, in planning actions or analyzing a visual scene. In this book the term is not used in relation to disorders of the production or decoding of speech (see "aphasiological disorder").

cognitive linguistics: linguistic theory based on the idea that major syntactical categories of language (such as time, space, and the subject-verb-object link) arise from invariables in the registers of perception and motor skills. There is no direct relation between cognitive linguistics and cognitive science.

cognitive science: theory that sees perception as functioning through separate mental modules, each processing fragmentary data from the real world.

communication disorder: dysfunction of exchange, apparent in symptoms such as avoidance of eye contact, absence of facial expressions, and lack of pointing, which show that the disorder of a child with language problems goes beyond language. Interpretations vary with schools of thought, one referring to deficiencies and another to the organization of defense mechanisms. Typical of the range of autistic disorders.

concrete play: rooted like figurative play, but unlike abstract play, in simulations of real human situations and activity, requiring interacting characters drawn from reality or fantasy.

connection between sensation and perception: in my usage, "sensation" means the effect of the outside world on the body or the sense organs; it is directly related to muscular tonus and posture of the body. "Perception" refers to the organizing of data received from the outside world so as to construct a coherent representation, which may then enable a subject to act upon the world. In ordinary children, sensation and perception are linked and in harmony. In the autistic child, sensation often prevails over perception, and the two are not linked.

consonantal skeleton: disposition of the consonants in a word that makes it possible to recognize the complete signifier and its meaning even when the vowels are missing, as in "c th d r l" (= "cathedral").

countables and uncountables: in linguistics, categories of nouns signifying things that can be counted (e.g., "a marble," "several marbles") as opposed to those that do not usually lend themselves to being counted, often referring to substances (e.g., "butter," "water," "wine"). Countable nouns can usually take the plural without changing their meaning, whereas plurals of uncountable nouns tend to mean a set of qualitatively different entities (e.g., "wines").

countertransference: term used in psychoanalysis for the assortment of feelings and sensations, agreeable and disagreeable, affectionate and disaffectionate, experienced by a therapist during a session in response to the material generated by the child. One must try to identify these feelings and sensations, not just to contain them but also to achieve a better understanding of what is going on in a child's ways of relating and playing.

décentrement: Piaget's term (meaning roughly "off-centering") denoting the ability to change one's point of view in the cognitive processing of a set of objects. One may safely say that any child who is capable of putting together sets of images first according to shape (round, square, and triangular) and then according to color (greens, reds, and blues) possesses this ability. The second of these operations presupposes the ability to ignore the first, to "off-center" the earlier criterion of classification and to opt for another way of organizing the material.

decontextualization: ability to use the same word to mean identical things in different situations or contexts. In so doing, a child frees him- or herself from the constraints imposed on the word by a particular context. This happens when a child can say "water" about what is in his beaker, what falls on his face when it rains, and what runs out of the bath tap. It means the child's use of the notion is no longer dependent on the situation in which the thing originally occurred. This is an ability that appears to be lacking in autistic children whose use of words is restricted to the context in which they first heard them.

depressive position: see page 164.

developmental pathology: study of disorders of the development of psychic, cognitive, and affective faculties in children. Different disciplines, such as pediatrics, social sciences, psychology, cognitive psychology, psychoanalysis, may arrive at markedly different theoretical interpretations of this sort of disorder. This is especially the case in the field of disorders of communication.

dismantling and dissociation: related terms, the first used in psychoanalysis, the second in cognitive science, for symptoms observed in children with an autistic spectrum disorder. Refers to a propensity to isolate each of the elements that should be associated in a process of perception, action, or interaction with someone else.

displacement: any slight variation or change introduced by a child into repetitive play, attesting to the fact that the game is not exactly replicated each time, as is the case with autistic stereotypy.

dissociation: see "dismantling."

disturbance of relationships: spectrum of instrumental and/or psychogenic disorders, including childhood psychosis, autism, and pervasive development disorders, theorized in different ways by different disciplines. I refer to this insofar as it is present in communication disorders. Though nonverbal, these disorders have implications for language, especially disorders of gesture and movement, facial expression during verbal exchange, and intonation.

drive: term used in psychoanalysis for the source of any psychic activity. Such activity arises from any lack or dissatisfaction that originates in the body but that, unlike mere internal excitation, has acceded to the register of the psyche, where it can be represented.

drowsy nanny: see page 78.

DSM-IV: the American Psychiatric Association's *Diagnostic and Statistical Manual of Mental Disorders*.

dysphasia: strictly linguistic disorder, unrelated to communication, affecting the development of language in children, either in its reception or its production; at its most serious, it may entail total absence of language production (audimutism).

dysphasic syndrome: disorder of children affected by dysphasia, manifested mainly in production or reception of language. A production disorder may be marked by nongrammatical language (verbs unconjugated, articles omitted); a reception disorder may entail faulty differentiation of close phonemes (both in production and in recognition). This may lead to a secondary disorder in the language actually produced by the child: poor identification of language addressed to the child results in faulty production, though the origin of the disorder is not strictly one of production.

echolalia: linguistic behavior typical of autistic disorders, entailing the repetition by the child of what has been said, echoing both the words and the intonation. Immediate echolalia is repetition without delay; in delayed echolalia, a statement uttered in a particular situation may be repeated several days later.

enunciative linguistics: French branch of linguistics, founded by Antoine Culioli following the lead of Émile Benveniste. It posits that speech content can be understood only by taking account of the position of the speaker, of the addressee, and of the situation in which the speaker makes the utterance (in particular the moment at which it is made). These factors constitute the "coordinates" of the enunciative act.

exchange: the setting, content, and circumstances of communication taking place between two individuals, particularly a child and an adult, whether a parent, a friend, or a therapist.

expressive disorder: specific dysphasic disorder that affects language production (e.g., telegraphic style).

eye contact: normally shows intentions, affects, or joint interest; in effective communication, necessarily combines with facial expressions of varying import (e.g., interest, surprise, pleasure, displeasure, expectation).

eye movements: in an exchange, usually enable an interlocutor to interpret something of a speaker's or addressee's interest and attention.

eyesight: scanning behavior that enables a subject to appreciate all aspects of a situation. Some children with minor neurological disorders have deficient scanning abilities. For example, a child who is asked to mark all the baby rabbit shapes on a large sheet of paper containing shapes of various other animals may not realize that she has missed the baby rabbits in a particular area of the sheet. This deficient scanning can sometimes be limited to situations where an "obstacle" is built in, for example, if one draws a line across a large sheet of paper, then marks a series of numbered points along the line and asks the child to link them up in order of size, a child with a visual disorder sensitive to this type of obstacle may stop linking up the points if at any time it is necessary to cross the line drawn on the paper.

figurative play: see "concrete play."

first-language acquisition: process whereby a child learns his or her native language (see chapter 11).

formatting games: an extension from the idea of formatting developed by Jerome Bruner, who used it to define games played by mother and infant (e.g, hide-and-seek, appearing/disappearing) in which joint attention and communication focused on the object of attention develop. The idea of formatting stresses the regularizing effect of such games on the setting and form of the exchange and its rules: relating to others, the rhythm of the alternations, the ways of showing or designating the objects used in the exchange. To my mind, formatting games also have an effect on the way children build up a model of what is entailed in an action, relations between container and contained, the animate and the inanimate, and so on.

frontal disorders: in adults, includes a number of symptoms related to a disorder of the brain's frontal lobes, remarkably similar to some of the symptomatology observed in autism.

functional imaging: technology that provides images of cerebral activity, enabling observation of zones of the brain in action, both in normal subjects and in subjects with particular disorders.

grammar words: also called functional words, these mark the grammatical links between lexical terms in a statement: articles, pronouns, auxiliary verbs, and sometimes inflections such as the "s" added to the third person singular of verbs in the present tense ("she drives") or to the plurals of countable nouns ("goats").

handedness: denotes the choice of either the right or the left hand as the dominant one in tasks requiring cooperation between both hands.

high-functioning autism: way of characterizing children on the autistic spectrum who, though they manifest symptoms related to communication with others, are able to function in society. Typical symptoms include difficulty in making eye contact and in taking account of someone else's interest and expectation in conversation, high-pitched voice, and flat or stilted intonation. See "Asperger's syndrome" and "pervasive developmental disorders."

hyperlexia: ability of some autistic children to read isolated words even though they are incapable of any oral production. Some children recognize only the letters; some can spell them out orally; others can understand them as well as spell them out. It is a "hyper" ability compared to the poor oral production. This symptom is of variable value in prognosis: it can indicate a progressive inaptitude for oral production, but the ability to read written words can sometimes lead to a measure of oral production.

ICD: the World Health Organization's *International Classification of Diseases (10th Revision)*.

individuation: psychic process that enables a subject to come to a feeling of being separate from his or her love object (usually the mother). In normal psychological development, this stage follows the initial one in which the child, having no self-contained or private mind distinct from the mother's, does not yet recognize himself as a completely separate being. Clearly, this sketchy definition does not imply that children who have not achieved individuation constantly see their mother as an extension of their own identity.

integrative alternation: see page 50.

intentional speech: see page 53.

intermodality: see page 201.

internal bodily sensations: various modes of proprioceptive awareness of one's own body (the tactile, the coenesthetic and kinesthetic, those relating to posture and balance) that give pleasant or unpleasant information on the state of the body in its relation to the outside world.

joint attention: state of communication between two people, generally child and adult, marking the inception of a possible exchange. Both share interest in an independent external object (for instance, a toy) which will become a focus of communication. Conditional on certain neurological skills, for instance, the child's ability to understand that the adult's interest in an object can be deduced from the direction in which the latter is looking or pointing.

lallation: production by children too young to talk, consisting of sequences of linked sounds whose phonology and intonations belong to the language they hear around them.

language delay: minor language disorder in young children which the therapist may expect to cease spontaneously. Nothing more than a return visit six to twelve months later to check on this may be required. Accurately distinguishing delay from slight dysphasia needing treatment can be difficult.

language disorder: general term that includes all and any problems of language, as opposed to communication disorders (see chapter 1).

language learning: process whereby children acquire the faculty of language and description of the stages through which they pass. This book focuses on disorders that affect this process (see chapter 11 for normal development).

language pathology: broadly speaking, all disorders of language and communication in children and adults. Strictly speaking, the term excludes disorders of communication, ranging from pervasive developmental disorders (PDD) and psychosis to autism, and means only those of language.

leucodystrophy: any of several genetically determined diseases (e.g., adrenoleukodystrophy) characterized by progressive degeneration of myelin in the brain, spinal cord, and peripheral nerves.

lexical words: terms with meaning content, generally entered in dictionaries. In "Jean eats an apple" the lexical words are "Jean," "eats," and "apple" ("an" being a grammar word).

lexico-referential categories: categories such as action or object. Within these categories there are subcategories that oppose verbs expressing actions and verbs expressing states, or human and nonhuman objects, or animate and inanimate objects.

linguistic disorder: see "language disorder."

linguistic pragmatics: theory deriving from the basic hypothesis that language and communication constitute a human activity that aims to impinge on an addressee by means other than direct violence. This theory construes speaking as action. However, though it is helpful in analyzing injunctive statements (orders and similar modes of address, including imperatives), it is barely compatible with the idea that language can produce a sharing of affect or shared pleasure without such a purpose.

logopedics: term used in French-speaking Switzerland and Belgium in the field of speech therapy. Implies more than a difference of word; the therapist's concern is for the child's language and development as distinct from questions of right or wrong use, or grammatical or ungrammatical expression.

macrocephaly: genetic disorder marked, among other things, by the fact that a subject's head is too large in proportion to the rest of the body.

mechanics of speech: my term for anything that entails the neurology of speech (including procedures of encoding and decoding the sound chain) as opposed to the symbolic dimension of speech and the way it helps a subject to organize his or her identity or representation of things in their absence.

mental lexicon: theoretical construct that helps explain the way a subject grasps the meaning of the words that make up a sentence and contrives to assemble a statement on the basis of an idea that he or she wishes to express. A mental lexicon is the way one imagines words are stored in the memory. Clearly, whatever one can say about such a subject is no more than a crude stab in the dark.

metapsychology: Freud's term for the hypotheses that underlie concepts in psychoanalysis (e.g., repression, wish fulfillment), dealing in particular with considerations germane to the duality of drives (life and death instincts, Eros and Thanatos).

metarepresentation: ability to relate a state of affairs, notably the behavior of an individual, to a cause that is not directly observable and that entails the implicit representation of another person. An example of a metarepresentation: you take someone's keys out of his pocket and put them in a box without his noticing what you are doing. He will therefore look for them in his pocket (and not in the box where you happen to know they are). Your recognition that he will look in his pocket and not in the box involves awareness of another's representation (he believes the keys are still in his pocket, because he did not see you take them out) and knowing the difference between that representation and what is a fact (I know the keys are in the box, because I saw them there).

mirror neurons: see chapter 13, "The Peanut and Babies Who Stick Out Their Tongues."

modularity: see page 201.

motor skills: include a child's ways of "living" in his or her body, as well as general movements or gross motor skills (e.g., running, jumping, climbing, catching a ball, throwing it back) and fine motor skills, including hand movements, the ability to take things between finger and thumb or to hold a pencil, and the ability to draw lines, to draw, and to write (see page 19).

motor program: complete repertory of actions needed to achieve a required result, such as getting a book down from a top shelf or coloring in a drawing of a house. Programs involve different stages, which may give rise to a range of disorders. Once learned, a program must be retained in memory and its execution must be regularly checked to gauge any disparity between the result achieved and the result aimed at in any of the stages.

mouth noises: made and identically repeated by some children with communication disorders; often mere sounds and not phonemes. They are the audible outcome of a sort of stereotyped action of the tongue, the lips, and the whole mouth and phonation apparatus. In less severe cases, it is at times possible to see them as having a meaning (in terms of the moment when they are made, for instance) and to observe some gradual diversification in them.

neurocognitive dysfunction: disorder of neurological origin that complicates any particular cognitive task (see two examples at "eyesight").

neurological apparatus: the brain in its functions of organizing and monitoring the range of cognitive tasks, whether linguistic or nonlinguistic.

neuropsychology of language: discipline that endeavors to establish the modules and functions that help us understand how the sound chain is encoded and decoded and to account for any malfunctions of these processes.

nonverbal communication: communication without spoken sounds, essentially hand movements and gestures, motioning with the torso or the head, and facial expressions, smiling, eye glances, and so on.

nonverbal signs: signs in the form of gestures and expressions (see "nonverbal communication").

notions: see page 209.

onomatopoeia: category of word whose signifier is linked to the referent or the situation in which it occurs, like "vroom," meaning a car or "splosh" for something falling in the water; the sound of the word imitating the sound of the phenomenon being referred to.

parlances: term referring to a child's different ways of speaking, or styles of speech, before language has become fully established and homogeneous; implies a development of language within distinct zones of activity, each zone corresponding to different activities or interests.

patient: in linguistics, noun phrase or equivalent identifying a person or thing having something done to them (e.g., "Augustina" in *Young Binks kissed Augustina*).

pedantic voice: affected tone of voice observed in some children with particular communication disorders, possibly a throwback to delayed echolalia (see definition) and a vestige of the adult voice that first spoke the words the child is now using.

peekaboo games: highly structured game of a type described by Bruner as formatting games (see definition), involving initial disappearance followed by the reappearance of the adult and the later disappearance followed by the reappearance of the child, helping children to construct the "there/not there" contrast, one of the essential lexico-referential categories.

pervasive developmental disorders: term used to define massive disorders in a child's development, sometimes akin to certain atypical forms of autism, though different from high-functioning autism or Asperger's syndrome (see definitions).

phoneme: smallest distinct sound unit in any given language.

phonologic-syntactic syndrome: see page 22.

pointing: has two basic modes, the proto-imperative (e.g., a child indicates an object that he wants to be given) and the proto-declarative (e.g., a child draws an adult's attention to something as the basis for an exchange, leading to joint attention). The latter form almost guarantees that the child is not autistic.

pragmatics disorder: term sometimes used for disorders of communication associated less with the content of statements produced than with the use made of the content and the mode of participation in exchange (e.g., the child takes no cognizance of the interlocutor's expectations in engaging in the exchange).

prelanguage communication: see "preverbal communication."

prelanguage disorders: disorders of preverbal communication, often indicative of autism or childhood psychosis.

preverbal communication: communication that relies on gesture, movement, facial expressions, and intonations (though intonation verges on the verbal, it is not yet segmental, unlike phonemes).

preverbal signifiers: see "preverbal communication" (and an example at "pointing").

primary thinking: Freud's term for a way of thinking via associations and impulses, as opposed to the "secondary process" of thought, which takes account of the constraints of reality.

production: covers anything related to the use of speech and the encoding of the sound chain.

profound dysphasia: particularly severe mode of dysphasia, usually depriving children of all language; most profound dysphasics are affected by a massive disorder of language reception that, by preventing them from recognizing the phonemes spoken to them, renders them incapable of speech.

proper nouns: names of persons or places, usually written with an initial capital, as opposed to common nouns.

proprioception: perceptions and sensations via which a subject experiences his or her own body and its spatial position; see "bodily sensations."

prosody: used here synonymously with "intonation."

protosignifiers: a child's first words, not necessarily belonging to adult vocabulary, expressing thought about things happening in the world (various affects, expressions of satisfaction or dissatisfaction).

psychic tension: state induced by any disparity between what one wants and what one has, or by any feeling of contradictory desires, to be resolved by an action that may be vocal.

psychoanalytical semiotherapy: my own coinage for what this book is about, the kind of work I do with children without language. The psychoanalytical part derives from my training as an analyst, which frames my way of understanding the children's acts and feelings and my own countertransference; the semiotherapy is my way of helping these children to produce signs (not necessarily language) in order to communicate with others.

psychomotor treatment: therapy based on the idea that relationships with others build on basic bodily posture prior to any communication through gesture or speech. It consists of various activities that involve general motor skills, with the aim of making children aware of their own bodies and the ways in which, notably in play, their relating to others affects their physical posture (muscle tone, attitude, movements).

"pure" language disorder: language disorder unrelated to any autistic or psychotic disorder of communication but still capable of having a marked effect on a child's psychic functioning.

receptive disorder: see page 23.

registers of intentionality: term expressing the degree of a child's awareness of any of his or her own acts or gestures and their meaning as signs. An act or gesture may be no more than an unintended reaction to the presence of an adult, and it may be the latter who reads meaning into it as a communicative sign and reshapes it as such for the child. There are gradations of intentionality between unintended reaction and deliberate communicative sign.

referentiality: use of language to indicate an object or an event via a lexical term, appearing significantly later in a child's development than is usually thought, early use of, say, "ball" expressing not the object but the ball game (throwing and catching) played with another person.

representation: very broad term, used in this work to mean whatever inner construction a child contrives to put upon anything real but not immediately perceptible or anything imaginary. Representation can be said to exist if psychic activity involves persons or things not actually present. Generally, communication requires a second order of representation consisting of an engagement with the mind of an interlocutor (the representation of someone else's representation).

ritual: repetition of a relatively unchanging sequence of actions or hand movements. Autistic stereotypy is a totally unchanging ritual.

same/not same: see "categorization."

scenario: set sequence of actions associated in the mind of a child with an object.

scenario games: mode of concrete play (see definition) as opposed to abstract play, in which either toy figures are made to mime situations (mother, father, baby) or the child mimes an action with, for example, a doll or a tea set.

secondary autism: sometimes differentiated from primary. In primary autism, the child is utterly cut off from exchange with others and appears not to know she is separate from the world of things and especially from her love object, her mother. In secondary autism, incipient differentiation can give the child a sense of being partly separate from the inert world and even from the love object, which can provoke fear of individuation and extremely violent reactions of anxiety and anger.

segmental communication: communication through speech in its complete phonological dimension, as opposed to sign language, facial expressions, or the use of the mere intonations of speech.

self-directed speech: see page 53.

semantic-pragmatic syndrome: way of defining the discourse of those who suffer from childhood psychosis, though not recognized by some authorities, who assimilate it to a "pure" disorder of language production, despite the fact that it has an effect on the organizing and uses of discourse rather than on the production of signifiers. May also be affected by a frontal disorder.

semiotic functioning: activity of a subject capable of transforming his or her acts into signs, such as when a child turns his tears into a show of displeasure for his mother or when a child in therapy grasps a segment of a ritualized scenario as meaning that a new segment, known to both partners in the exchange, is about to follow.

semiotics: as opposed to linguistics, which is the study of meaning organized by signs made solely of language, this is the science of the making of signs, with special focus on qualitative differences between different types of signs and signifiers used by a subject (see "registers of intentionality").

severe expressive syndrome: purely linguistic syndrome that affects production of the sound chain.

side-by-side play: see page 87.

sign: made from the association of two elements: a material element, constituting the signifier, produced by the initiator of exchange, meant to be received by its addressee, and standing for a mental content which constitutes the signified.

signified: see "sign."

signifier: see "sign."

sign language: used by the deaf and dumb, containing signifiers made exclusively of hand movements and facial expressions.

sound contour: that which enables the brain to recognize a spoken word, the type of ability affected by a receptive disorder.

speech disorder: distinct from disorders of communication and personality.

speech mechanism: term for the different modules and functions identified by neurology, neuropsychology, and aphasiology as being responsible for the encoding and decoding of the sound chain.

stereotypy: repetitive movement made by an autistic child in the presence of someone else, as though to look at ease and vent a feeling of agitation; also perceptible in normal subjects, (e.g. twiddling one's thumbs in an idle or slack moment).

Sturge-Weber's syndrome: neurological disorder akin in certain respects to autistic symptomatology.

suprasegmental communication: element of verbal communication supplied by intonation and the melody of speech, crucial, for example, in questions; "You want to eat" may be a meaningless statement unless a rising intonation shows that a question is being asked.

symbolic equation: concept proposed by Hanna Segal for the use of signs made by some psychotic patients, for whom the sign "equals" the thing and any procedure done with the sign means a procedure done with the thing.

symbolization: the way a subject is able to "think his thoughts," as Wilfred Bion puts it, how a subject contrives to represent his own way of producing representation and how he figures the disparity between what he desires and reality, or between what he is thinking and what he thinks someone else is thinking. Full symbolization implies the existence of a theory of mind (see definition) and acess to metarepresentation, which implies recourse to the depressive position.

syntactical words: see page 194.

telegraphic style: mode of speaking in some children with a disorder of production, wholly or partly lacking syntactical words, after the manner of a telegram, for example, "Impossible come tomorrow" instead of "I am unable to come tomorrow."

theme and rheme: see page 92.

theory of mind: term used by David Premack in his work on the behavior of chimpanzees, positing that a subject has a representation that enables him to see that others also have representations of the external world which help account for their actions. To have a theory of mind is to have a representation of others' representations (see "metarepresentation"). This term has since been used by Uta Frith and S. Baron-Cohen to account for autistic children's inability to anticipate other people's behaviors and attitudes.

thought control: see page 84.

topic and comment: see page 92.

turn-taking: see page 42.

verbal auditory agnosia: disorder of perception of speech in which the subject cannot distinguish between the different phonemes of what is being said. Not a form of deafness, in that perception of the sounds is not affected; hearing of noises and music may also be intact. As in any agnosia, the subject is unaware of it as a disorder.

vocabulary explosion: qualitative leap in vocabulary development, usually occurring between the ages of eighteen months and two years, when the child may acquire several new words every day.

voicing: a term I use for the uttering of any meaningful sound.

West's syndrome: neurological disorder akin in certain respects to autistic symptomatology.

Bibliography

(Dates are not necessarily those of first publication but those of the editions used.)

Language Disorders

Aimard, P. *Les Troubles du langage chez l'enfant*. Paris: Presses universitaires de France, 1984.

Ajuriaguerra, J. de. "Speech disorders in childhood." *Speech language and communication*, ed. E. C. Carterette, vol. 3, 117–140. Los Angeles: University of California Press, 1966.

Ajuriaguerra, J. de. "Organisation psychologique et troubles du développement du langage." In J. de Ajuriaguerra et al., *Problèmes de psycho-linguistique*, 109–142. Paris: Presses universitaires de France, 1963.

Ajuriaguerra, J. de, S. Borel-Maisonny, R. Diatkine, R. Narlian, and M. Sambak. "Le groupe des audimutités." *La Psychiatrie de l'enfant* 1, 1: 6–62. Paris: Presses universitaires de France, 1958.

Ajuriaguerra, J. de, R. Diatkine, and D. Kalmanson. "Les troubles du développement du langage au cours des états psychotiques précoces." *La Psychiatrie de l'enfant* 2, 1: 1–65. Paris: Presses universitaires de France, 1959.

Ajuriaguerra, J. de, et al. "Organisation et désorganisation du langage chez l'enfant." In J. de Ajuriaguerra, *Manuel de psychiatrie de l'enfant*, 329–353. Paris: Masson, 1970.

Ajuriaguerra, J. de, et al. "Évolution et pronostic de la dysphasie chez l'enfant." *La Psychiatrie de l'enfant* 8, 2: 391–452. Paris: Presses universitaires de France, 1965.

Bierwisch, M., and E. Weigl. "Neuropsychology and linguistics." *Cortex* 24 (1970): 13–32.

Bishop, D. V. M. "Autism, Asperger's syndrome and semantic-pragmatic disorder: Where are the boundaries?" *Journal of Disorders of Communication* 24 (1989): 107–121.

Boubli, M. "Les mots dans la bouche." In D. Anzieu, G. Haag, S. Tisseron, G. Lavallée, M. Boubli, and J. Lassègue, *Les Contenants de pensée*, 127–144. Paris: Dunod, 1995.

Boubli, M. "Émergence du langage au cours d'une psychothérapie d'enfant." In *Pulsions, représentations, langage*, ed. M. Pinol-Douriez, 135–160. Lausanne: Delachaux et Niestlé, 1997.

Boubli-Elbez, M. "La bouche: de la sensorialité au langage." Doctoral diss., Université de Provence, 1995.

Bresson, M.-F. "L'état actuel des recherches sur les dysphasies." *Les Textes du centre Alfred Binet, Dysphasies* 11 (décembre 1987): 25–51.

Chiat, S., J. Law, and J. Marshall, eds. *Language Disorders in Children and Adults: Psycholinguistic Approaches to Therapy*. London: Whurr, 1977.

Christe, R., M. M. Christe-Luterbacher, and P. Luquet. *La Parole troublée*. Paris: Presse universitaires de France, 1997.

Conti-Ramsden, G., and S. Friel-Patti. "Mothers' discourse adjustments to language-impaired and non-language-impaired children." *Journal of Speech and Hearing Disorders* 48 (1983): 360–367.

Cramblitt, N. S., and G. M. Siegel. "Verbal environment of a language-impaired child." *Journal of Speech and Hearing Disorders* 42 (1977): 474–482.

Danon-Boileau, L. "La dysphasie : un agrégat disparate de 'savoir-dire' multiples." In *Le Français et ses usages à l'oral et à l'écrit*, ed. K. Boucher. Paris: Presses de la Sorbonne Nouvelle, 2001.

Danon-Boileau, L. *The Silent Child*. Oxford: Oxford University Press, 2001.

Diatkine, R. "Essai sur les dysphasies." *Les Textes du centre Alfred Binet, Dysphasies* 11 (décembre 1987): 1–16.

Diatkine, R. "La place de l'étude du langage dans l'examen psychiatrique de l'enfant." In *Traité de psychiatrie de l'enfant et de l'adolescent*, t. 1, ed. S. Lebovici, R. Diatkine, and M. Soulé, 385–391. Paris: Presses universitaires de France, 1985.

Diatkine, R. "Les troubles de la parole et du langage." In *Traité de psychiatrie de l'enfant et de l'adolescent*, t. 2, ed. S. Lebovici, R. Diatkine, and M. Soulé, 385–423. Paris: Presses universitaires de France, 1985.

Diatkine, R., and P. Denis. "Les psychoses infantiles." In *Traité de psychiatrie de l'enfant et de l'adolescent*, t. 2, ed. S. Lebovici, R. Diatkine, and M. Soulé, 185–224. Paris: Presses universitaires de France, 1985.

Garrett, M. F. "The analysis of sentence production." In *Psychology of Learning and Motivation*, vol. 9, ed. G. Bower, 133–177. New York: Academic Press, 1975.

Gelbert, G. *Lire, c'est aussi écrire*. Paris: Editions Odile Jacob, 1998.

Gérard, C.-L. *L'Enfant dysphasique*. Paris: Éditions universitaires, 1991.

Giroire, J.-M. "L'aphasie de l'enfant et ses formes limites." In *La Lecture, Psychologie et neuropsychologie*, t. 2, ed. N. Zavialoff, 162–168. Paris: L'Harmattan, 1990.

Houzel, D. Introduction au colloque "Genèse et psychopathologie du langage chez l'enfant" (Brest, mai 1993). *Neuropsychiatrie de l'enfance et de l'adolescence* 32–10/11: 477–491.

Jackson, J. H. *Selected Writings*, ed. J. Taylor. London: Staples Press, 1931.

Lebovici, S., et al. "À propos des observations des calculateurs de calendrier." *La Psychiatrie de l'enfant* 9, 2: 341–396.

Leonard, L. B., R. G. Schwartz, K. Chapman, L. Rowan, P. Prelock, B. Terrel, A. Weiss, and C. Messick. "Early lexical acquisition in children with specific language impairment." *Journal of Speech and Hearing Research* 25 (1982): 554–564.

Locke, J. L. "The influence of speech perception in the phonologically disordered child." *Journal of Speech and Hearing Disorders* 45, 4 (1980): 431–468.

Luria, A. R. *Higher Cortical Functions in Man*. London: Tavistock, 1966.

Mazeau, M. *Dysphasies, troubles mnésiques, syndrome frontal chez l'enfant*. Paris: Masson, 1997.

Minshew, N. J., G. Goldstein, and D. J. Siegel. "Speech and language in high-functioning autistic individuals." *Neuropsychology* 3, 2 (1995): 255–261.

Rapin, I., and D. A. Allen. "Developmental language disorders." In *Handbook of Neuropsychology of Language*, vol. 7, *Child Neurobiology*, ed. Sj. Segalowitz and I. Rapin, 111–137. New York: Elsevier Science Publishers, 1992.

Rapin, I., and D. A. Allen. "Developmental dysphasia and autism in preschool children: characteristics and subtypes." *Proceedings of the First International Symposium on Specific Speech and Language Disorders in Children* (1987): 20–35.

Rapin, I., and D. A. Allen. "Developmental language disorders: nosologic considerations." In *Neuropsychology of Language, Reading and Spelling*, ed. U. Kirk, 155–184. New York: Academic Press, 1983.

Rondal, J., and X. Séron. *Troubles du langage, diagnostic et rééducation*. Bruxelles: Mardaga, 1982.

Weck, G. de. *Troubles du langage, perspectives pragmatiques et discursives*. Genève: Delachaux et Niestlé, 1995.

Autism (works with a cognitive science approach)

Adolphs, R., D. Tranei, and A. R. Damasio. "The human amygdala in social judgment." *Nature* 393 (1998): 470–474.

Adrien, J.-L., N. Rossignol, C. Barthélemy, and D. Sauvage. "Évaluation neuropsychologique d'un enfant autiste de bon niveau. À propos de l'hypothèse frontale dans l'autisme." *Approche Neuropsychologique des apprentissages chez l'enfant* 5 (1993): 155–161.

Baron-Cohen, S. "Theory of mind and autism: a fifteen-year review." In *Understanding Other Minds: Perspectives from Developmental Cognitive Neuroscience*, ed. S. Baron-Cohen, H. Tager-Flusberg, and D. J. Cohen, 2nd ed., 3–20. Oxford: Oxford University Press, 2000.

Baron-Cohen, S. *Mindblindness: An essay on Autism and Theory of Mind*. Cambridge, Mass.: Bradford, MIT Press, 1995.

Baron-Cohen, S., A. M. Leslie, and U. Frith. "Does the autistic child have a 'theory of mind'?" *Cognition* 21 (1985): 37–46.

Bursztejn, C., and A. Gras-Vincendon. "La 'théorie de l'esprit': un modèle de développement de l'intersubjectivité?" *Neuropsychiatrie enfance et adolescence* 49 (2001): 35–41.

Damasio, A. R., and R. G. Maurer. "A neurological model for childhood autism." *Archives Neurologiques* 33 (1978): 777–786.

Dennett, D. C. *Consciousness Explained*. Boston: Little, Brown, 1991.

Fadiga, L., G. Fogassi, G. Pavese, V. Gallese, and A. Goldman. "Mirror neurons and the simulation theory of mind-reading." *Trends in Cognitive Sciences* 2 (1998): 493–501.

Fogassi L., V. Gallese, L. Fadiga, and G.Rizzolatti. "Premotor cortex and the recognition of motor actions." *Cognitive Brain Research* 3 (1996): 131–141.

Frith, U. "L'autisme." *Pour la science* 190 (août 1993): 66–73.

Frith, U. *Autism: Explaining the Enigma*. Oxford: Basil Blackwell, 1989.

Jeannerod, M., M. A. Arbib, G. Rizzolatti, and I. Sakata. "Grasping objects: The cortical mechanisms of visuomotor transformation." *Trends in Neurosciences* 18 (1995): 314–320.

Kanner, L. "Autistic disturbances of affective contact." *Nervous Child* 2 (1943): 217–250.

Merians, A. S., M. Clark, H. Poizner, B. Macauley, L. J. Gonzalez-Rothi, and K. Heilman. "Visual-imitative dissociation apraxia." *Neuropsychologia* 35 (1997): 1483–1490.

Mottron, L., J. Burack, J. E. Stauder, and P. Robaey. "Perceptual processing among high-functioning persons with autism." *Journal of Child Psychology and Psychiatry* 40 (1999): 203–212.

Ozanoff, S., and D. L. Strayer. "Inhibitory function in non-retarded children with autism." *Journal of Autism & Developmental Disorders* 27, 1 (1997): 59–77.

Premack, D. "Upgrading a Mind." In *Talking Minds*, ed. T. G. Bever, J. M. Carroll, and L. A. Miller, 181–208. Cambridge, Mass.: MIT Press, 1984.

Rizzolatti, G., and M. A. Arbib. "Language within our grasp." *Trends in Neurosciences* 21 (1998): 188–194.

Rizzolatti, G., L. Fadiga, G. Fogassi, and V. Gallese. "Resonance behavior and mirror neurons." *Archives italiennes de biologie* 137 (1999): 85–100.

Veneziano, E., M. H. Plumet, C. Tardif, and S. Cupello. "A comparative study of conflict negotiation in autistic and control group children varying in verbal mental age." *Xth European Conference on Developmental Psychology*, Uppsala, Sweden, 2001.

Autism (psychoanalytical works)

Bick, E. "The experience of the skin in early object relations." *International Journal of Psychoanalysis* 49 (1968): 484–486.

Bion, W. R. "A theory of thinking." *International Journal of Psychoanalysis* 43 (1962): 306–310.

Bion, W. R. "Attacks on linking." *International Journal of Psychoanalysis* 40 (1959): 308–315.

Bion, W. R. "Language and the schizophrenic." In *New Directions in Psycho-Analysis*, ed. M. Klein, P. Heimann, and R. E. Money-Kyrle, 220–239. London: Tavistock, 1955.

Castoriadis-Aulagnier, P. *La Violence de l'interprétation. Du pictogramme à l'énoncé.* Paris: Presses universitaires de France, 1975.

Diatkine, R. "L'autisme infantile précoce : un point de vue psychanalytique en 1993." *La Psychiatrie de l'enfant* 36, 2 (1993): 363–412.

Diatkine, R., and J. Simon. *La Psychanalyse précoce.* Paris: Presses universitaires de France, 1972.

Haag, G. "De la sensorialité aux ébauches de pensée chez les enfants autistes." *Revue internationale de psychopathologie* 3 (1991): 51–63.

Haag, G. "Autisme infantile précoce et phénomènes autistiques, réflexions psychanalytiques." *Psychanalyse de l'enfant et de l'adolescent* 25 (1984): 293–355.

Hochman, J. *Pour soigner l'enfant autiste.* Paris: Éditions Odile Jacob, 1997.

Hochman, J. "L'autisme infantile, déficit ou défense." In *Soigner, éduquer l'enfant autiste*, ed. P. Parquet, C. Bursztejn, and B. Golse. Paris: Masson, 1989.

Houzel, D. "Pensée et stabilité structurelle. À propos des théories post-kleiniennes de l'autisme infantile." *Revue internationale de psychopathologie* 3 (1991): 97–112.

Houzel, D. "Le monde tourbillonnaire de l'autisme." *Lieux de l'enfance* 3 (1985): 169–183.

Klein, M. "Mourning and its relation to Manic-Depressive states," *International Journal of Psycho Analysis* 21 (1940), reprinted in *Contribution to Psycho-analysis*, 311–338. London: Hogarth Press and Institute of Psycho-analysis, 1950.

Lebovici, S., and D.-J. Duché. "Le concept d'autisme et de psychose chez l'enfant. Coup d'œil sur leur histoire." In *Autisme et psychoses de l'enfant*, ed. P. Mazet and S. Lebovici, 9–19. Paris: Presses universitaires de France, 1990.

Mahler, M. *On Human Symbiosis and the Vicissitudes of Individuation*. New York: International Universities Press, 1968.

Mazet, P., and S. Lebovici, eds. *Autisme et psychoses de l'enfant*. Paris: Presses universitaires de France, 1990.

Meltzer, D. "The psychology of autistic states and post autistic mentality." In D. Meltzer, J. Bremner, S. Hoxter, D. Weddell, and I. Wittenberg. *Explorations in Autism*. Strath Tay, Perthshire, Scotland: Clunie Press, 1991.

Misès, R. *Les Pathologies limites de l'enfance*. Paris: Presses universitaires de France, 1990.

Racamier, P.-C. "Les paradoxes des schizophrènes." *Revue française de psychanalyse* 42 (1978): 877–969.

Ribas, D. "Chronique de l'intrication et de la désintrication pulsionnelle." *Bulletin de la société psychanalytique de Paris* 62 (nov.-déc. 2001): 1689–1797.

Ribas, D. *Un cri obscur, l'énigme des enfants autistes*. Paris: Calmann-Lévy, 1992.

Ribas, D. "Repérages métapsychologiques dans l'autisme infantile." In *Autismes de l'enfance*, ed. R. Perron and D. Ribas, 129–147. Paris: Presses universitaires de France, 1984.

Tustin, F. *The Protective Shell in Children and Adults*. London: Karnac Books, 1990.

Tustin, F. *Autistic States in Children*. London: Routledge and Kegan Paul, 1981.

Tustin, F. *Autism and Childhood Psychosis*. London: Hogarth, 1972.

Winnicott, D. W. *Playing and Reality*, London: Tavistock, 1971.

Winnicott, D. W. *Collected Papers: Through Pediatrics to Psychoanalysis*. London: Tavistock, 1957.

Linguistics and Psychoanalysis

Anzieu, D. *Le Moi-peau*. Paris: Dunod, 1995.

Anzieu, D. "Les signifiants formels et le Moi-peau." In D. Anzieu, D. Houzel, A. Missenard, M. Enriquez, A. Anzieu, J. Guillaumin, J. Doron, E. Lecourt, and T. Nathan, *Les Enveloppes psychiques*, 1–22. Paris: Dunod, 1987.

Anzieu, D. "Au fond de Soi, le toucher." *Revue française de psychanalyse* 48 (1984): 1385–1398.

Anzieu, D., et al. *Psychanalyse et langage*. Paris: Dunod, 1977.

Danon-Boileau, L. *Le Sujet de l'énonciation*. Paris: Ophrys, 1984.

Freud, S. "On Negation." In *The Standard Edition of the Complete Psychological Works*, vol. XIX. London: Hogarth Press, 1961.

Freud, S. "The Unconscious." In *The Standard Edition of the Complete Psychological Works*, vol. XIV. London: Hogarth Press, 1957.

Freud, S. "Beyond the Pleasure Principle." In *The Standard Edition of the Complete Psychological Works*, vol. XVIII. London: Hogarth Press, 1955.

Green, A. "Le langage dans la psychanalyse." In *Langages, IIIᵉ rencontres psychanalytiques d'Aix-en-Provence*, 19–250. Paris: Les Belles Lettres, 1983.

Luquet, P. "Langage, pensée et structure psychique." In *Rapport du 47ᵉ congrès des psychanalystes de langue française des pays romans* (1987).

Pichon, E. "La grammaire en tant que mode d'exploration de l'inconscient." *L'Évolution psychiatrique* 1 (1925): 237–257.

Rosolato, G. "Destin du signifiant." *Nouvelle revue de psychanalyse* 30 (1984): 139–170.

Segal, H. "Notes on symbol formation." *International Journal of Psychoanalysis* 31 (1957): 268–278.

Spitz, R. A. *Le Non et le Oui.* Paris: Presses universitaires de France, 1973.

Winnicott, D. W. *Playing and Reality.* London: Tavistock, 1975.

Language Acquisition

Bacri, N. "L'intelligibilité du langage enfantin : intonation et compréhension de la parole." In *Le Langage, Construction et actualisation*, ed. M. Moscato and G. Piéraut-Le Bonniec, 81–99. Rouen: Publications de l'université de Rouen, 98, 1984.

Bates, E., ed. *The Emergence of Symbols: Cognition and Communication in Infancy.* New York: Academic Press, 1979.

Bloom, L. ed. *Readings in Language Development.* New York: Wiley, 1978.

Bloom, L. *One Word at a Time: The Use of Single Word Utterances before Syntax.* The Hague: Mouton, 1973.

Boysson-Bardies, B. de. *Comment la parole vient aux enfants.* Paris: Éditions Odile Jacob, 1996.

Bresson, F. "Phylogenèse et ontogenèse du langage." In *Le Langage, Construction et actualisation*, ed. M. Moscato and G. Piéraut-Le Bonniec, 19–38. Rouen: Publications de l'université de Rouen, 98, 1989.

Brigaudiot, M., and C. Nicolas. "Les « Premiers Mots »." Doctoral diss., Université Paris-VII, 1990.

Bronckart, J.-P., P. Marieu, M. Siguan-Soler, H. Sinclair de Zwart, T. Slama-Cazacu, and A. Tabouret-Keller. *La Genèse de la parole.* Paris: Presses universitaires de France, 1977.

Brown, R. *A First Language, the Early Stages.* Cambridge, Mass.: Harvard University Press, 1973.

Bruner, J. S. *The Culture of Education.* Cambridge Mass.: Harvard University Press, 1996.

Bruner, J. S. *Child's Talk: Learning to Use Language.* New York: Norton, 1983.

Bulher, K. "Les lois générales d'évolution dans le langage de l'enfant." *Journal de psychologie* 23, 6 (1926): 597–607.

Clark, E. V. *The Lexicon in Acquisition*. Cambridge: Cambridge University Press, 1993.

Dore, J. "Holophrases, speech acts and language universals." *Journal of Child Language* 2 (1975): 21–40.

François, F., D. François, E. Sabeau-Jouannet, and M. Sourdot. *La Syntaxe de l'enfant avant cinq ans*. Paris: Larousse, 1976.

François, F., C. Hudelot, E. Sabeau-Jouannet, and M. Sourdot. *Conduites linguistiques chez le jeune enfant*. Paris: Presses universitaires de France, 1984.

Golinkoff, R., ed. *The Transition from Prelinguistic to Linguistic Communication*. Hillsdale, N.J.: Erlbaum, 1983.

Grégoire, A. *L'Apprentissage du langage, les deux premières années*. 2 vols. Liège: Bibliothèque de la Faculté des lettres, 1937, 1947.

Halliday, M. A. *Learning How to Mean: Exploration in the Development of Language*. London: Edward Arnold, 1975.

Karmiloff-Smith, A. *A Functional Approach to Child Language*. Cambridge: Cambridge University Press, 1979.

Konopczynski. G. "Le langage émergent : comment la mélodie devient intonation entre 8 et 24 mois." In *La Lecture, Psychologie et neuropsychologie*, t. 1, ed. N. Zavialoff, 329–341. Paris: L'Harmattan, 1990.

Menyuk, P. *The Acquisition and Development of Language*. New Jersey: Prentice Hall, 1971.

Moes, E. J. "The nature of representation and the development of consciousness. Language in infancy: a criticism of Moore and Meltzoff's neo-Piagetian approach." Paper presented at the International Conference on Infant Studies, New Haven, Conn., 1980.

Morgenstern, A. "L'Enfant apprenti-énonciateur." Doctoral diss., Université Paris-III, 1995.

Moscato, M. and G. Piéraut-Le Bonniec, eds. *Le Langage, Construction et actualisation*. Rouen: Publications de l'université de Rouen, 98, 1984.

Nelson, K. "Structure and strategy in learning to talk." *Monographs of the Society for Research in Child Development* 48 (149): 1973.

Nicolas-Jeantoux, C. *Juliette apprend à parler entre 12 et 24 mois*. Paris: Masson, 1980.

Slobin, D. I. "Universal and particular in the acquisition of language." In *Language Acquisition: The State of the Art*, ed. E. Wanner and L. R. Gleitman, 123–170. Cambridge: Cambridge University Press, 1982.

Symposium de l'Association de psychologie scentifique de langue française. *La Genèse de la parole*. Paris: Presses universitaires de France, 1977.

Veneziano, E. "Interaction, conversation et acquisition du langage dans les trois premières années." In *L'Acquisition du langage*, vol. I, *L'Émergence du langage*, ed. M. Kail and M. Fayol, 231–265. Paris: Presses universitaires de France, 2000.

Early Abilities

Bertoncini, J., and Boysson-Bardies, B. de. "La perception et la production de la parole avant deux ans." In *L'Acquisition du langage*, vol. I, ed. M. Kail and M. Fayol, 95–136. Paris: Presses universitaires de France, 2000.

Field, T. M. and R. Woodson, R, Greenberg, D. Cohen. "Discrimination and imitation of facial expressions by neonates." *Science* 218 (1982): 179–181.

Golinkoff. R., ed. *The Transition from Prelinguistic to Linguistic Communication*. Hillsdale, N.J.: Erlbaum, 1983.

Huber, G. "Intentionnalité et scénario dans les sciences cognitives et la psychanalyse." In *Penser-Apprendre. La cognition chez l'enfant. Les troubles de l'apprentissage. La prise en charge*. Les Colloques de Bobigny, 130–135. Paris: Eshel, 1988.

Kuhl, P., and A. Meltzoff. "The bimodal perception of speech in infancy." *Science* 218 (1982): 1138–1141.

MacKain, K., M. Studdert-Kennedy, S. Spicker, and D. N. Stern. "Infant intermodal speech perception is a left-hemisphere function." *Science* 219 (1983): 1347–1349.

Mehler, J., and E. Dupoux. *Naître humain*. Paris: Editions Odile Jacob, 1990.

Mother-Child Interactions

Bowlby, J. *Attachement et perte*. 3 vols. Paris: Presses universitaires de France, 1978.

Bruner, J. S. "Contexts and formats." In *Le Langage, Construction et actualisation*, ed. M. Moscato and G. Piéraut-Le Bonniec, 81–99. Rouen: Publications de l'université de Rouen, 98, 1984.

Burd, A. P., and A. E. Milewski. "Matching of facial gestures by young infants: Imitation or releasers?" Paper presented at the Meeting of the Society for Research in Child Development, Boston, 1981.

DeCasper, A. J., and W. P. Fifer. "Of human bonding: Newborns prefer their mother's voice." *Science* 208 (1980): 1174–1176.

Lebovici, S. *Le Nourrisson, la mère et le psychanalyste : les interactions précoces*. Paris: Éditions Bayard, 1999.

Pinol-Douriez, M. *Bébé agi-Bébé, actif*. Paris: Presses universitaires de France, 1984.

Scaife, M., and J. S. Bruner. "The capacity for joint visual attention in the infant." *Nature* 253 (1975): 256–266.

Stern, D. N. *The Interpersonal World of the Infant: A View from Psychoanalysis and Developmental Psychology*. New York: Basic Books, 1985.

Trevarthen, C. "Communication and co-operation in early infancy: a description of primary subjectivity." In *Before Speech: The Beginning of Interpersonal Communication*, ed. M. Bullowa, 321–347. Cambridge: Cambridge University Press, 1979.

Trevarthen, C., and K. J. Aitken. "Brain development, infant communication and empathy disorders: intrinsic factors in child mental health." *Development and Psychopathology* 6 (1994): 597–633.

Van Der Straten, A. *Premiers gestes, premiers mots : formes précoces de communication*. Paris: Bayard Centurion, 1991.

Child Psychology

Bresson, F. "Les fonctions de représentation et de communication." In *Psychologie*, Encyclopédie de la Pléiade, ed. J. Piaget and P. J.-P. Bronckart, 933–982. Paris: Gallimard, 1987.

Buhler, K. *The Mental development of the Child*. London: Kegan Paul, 1930 (= English translation of *Die geistige Entwicklung des Kindes*. Jena: G. Fischer, 1930).

Darwin, C. *The Expression of the Emotions in Man and Animals*. London: John Murray, 1872.

Malrieu, P. "Langage et représentation." In *La Genèse de la parole*, Symposium de l'Association de psychologie scentifique de langue française, 87–136. Paris: Presses universitaires de France, 1977.

Piaget, J. *La Formation du symbole chez l'enfant. Neuchâtel*: Delachaux et Niestlé, 1959.

Spitz, R. *The First Year of Life: A Psychoanalytic Study of Normal and Deviant Object Relation*. New York: International Universities Press, 1965.

Spitz, R. *On the Genesis of Human Communication*. New York: International Universities Press, 1957.

Vygotsky, L. S. *La Pensée et le langage*. Paris: Éditions Sociales, 1985.

Wallon, H. *L'Évolution psychologique de l'enfant*. Paris: Armand Colin, 1941.

Zazzo, R. *Reflets de miroir et autres doubles*. Paris: Presses universitaires de France, 1993.

General Linguistics, Philosophy of Language, Cognition

Apotheloz, D., and J.-B. Grize, eds. *Langage, processus cognitifs et genèse de la communication*. Travaux du centre de recherches sémiologiques de l'université de Neuchâtel, 54, 1987.

Austin, J. L. *How to Do Things with Words*. Oxford: Clarendon Press, 1962.

Bally, C. *Linguistique générale et linguistique française*. Berne: Francke, 1932.

Benveniste, E. *Problèmes de linguistique générale*, vol. 2. Paris: Gallimard, 1974.

Benveniste, E. *Problèmes de linguistique générale*, vol. 1. Paris: Gallimard, 1966.

Brunot, F. *La Pensée et la langue*. Paris: Masson, 1922.

Buhler, K. *Theory of Language, The Representational Function of Language*. Amsterdam/Philadelphia: John Benjamins, 1934.

Cassirer, E. *Philosophy of Symbolic Forms*. New Haven: Yale University Press, 1953–1957.

Culioli, A. *Pour une linguistique de l'énonciation*, vol. 1, *Opérations et représentations*. Paris: Ophrys, 1990.

Damourette, J., and E. Pichon. *Des mots à la pensée. Essai de grammaire de la langue française*. Paris: Éditions d'Artrey, 1911–1927.

Fodor, J. *The Modularity of Mind: an Essay on Faculty Psychology*. Cambridge, Mass.: MIT Press, 1983.

Fogassi, L., V. Gallese, L. Fadiga, and G. Rizzolati. "Neurons Responding to the Sight of Goal-Directed Hand-Arm Actions in the Parietal Area PF (7b) of the Macaque Monkey." *Soc. Neurosci. Abstracts* 257, 5 (1998): 654.

Halliday, M. A. K. *Explorations in the Functions of Language*. London: Edward Arnold, 1973.

Lakoff, G. *Women, Fire and Dangerous Things*. Chicago: University of Chicago Press, 1987.

Lakoff, G., and M. Johnson. *Metaphors We Live By*. Chicago: University of Chicago Press, 1980.

Langacker, R. W. *Cognitive Linguistics*, vol. I, 1–1. New York: Mouton de Gruyter, 1990.

Langacker, R. W. *Foundations of Cognitive Grammar*, vol. I. Stanford: Stanford University Press, 1987.

McNeill, D. *Language and Gesture*. Cambridge: Cambridge University Press, 2000.

Morel, M.-A., and Danon-Boileau, L. *Grammaire de l'intonation, l'exemple du français*. Paris: Ophrys, 1998.

Ninio, J. *L'Empreinte des sens*. Paris: Editions Odile Jacob, 1989.

Peirce, C. S. *Collected Papers*. Cambridge, Mass.: Harvard University Press, 1958.

Rosch, E. "Human categorization." In *Studies in Cross-cultural Psychology*, ed. N. Warren, 1–72. London: Academic Press, 1977.

Saussure, F. de. *Cours de linguistique générale*. Paris: Payot, 1972.

Vendler, Z. *Linguistics in Philosophy*. Ithaca: Cornell University Press, 1967.

Werner, H., and B. Kaplan. *Symbol Formation*. New York: Wiley, 1963.

Whorf, B. L. *Language, Thought and Reality: Selected Writings of Benjamin Lee Whorf*, ed. J. B. Carroll. Cambridge, Mass.: MIT Press, 1967.

Wierzbicka, A. *Lexicography and Conceptual Analysis*. Ann Arbor: Karoma, 1985.

Wittgenstein, L. *Philosophical Investigations*, New York: Macmillan, 1953.

Yau, S.-C. *Création gestuelle et débuts du langage. Création de langues gestuelles chez les sourds isolés*. Paris: Langages croisés, 1992.

Index